RACHAELE
HAMBLETON

PART-TIME
WORKING
MUMMY

A PATCHWORK LIFE

Tales of **Heartache**,
Hope and **Humour**
for Every Kind of Family

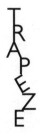

TRAPEZE

An Orion Paperback

First published in Great Britain in 2018
by Trapeze
This paperback edition published in 2019
By Trapeze, an imprint of The Orion Group Ltd,
Carmelite House, 50 Victoria Embankment,
London EC4Y 0DZ

An Hachette UK company

1 3 5 7 9 10 8 6 4 2

A CIP catalogue record for this book is available
from the British Library.

ISBN (Paperback): 978 1 409 18425 6

Typeset by Input Data Services Ltd, Somerset

Printed and bound by CPI Group (UK) Ltd, Croydon, CR0 4YY

The Orion Publishing Group's policy is to use papers that
are natural, renewable and recyclable products and
made from wood grown in sustainable forests. The logging
and manufacturing processes are expected to conform to
the environmental regulations of the country of origin.

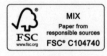

www.orionbooks.co.uk

PART-TIME WORKING MuMMY

For Betsy

Thank you
for showing me
what it feels like to fall in love.

Thank you for always giving me a reason
to fight when there were times I felt like giving up.

Thank you for making me see I wanted to make
lots more tiny humans just like you, because there
is no greater feeling than being a momma.

CONTENTS

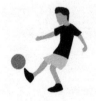

BETSY

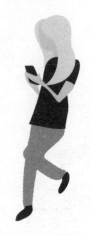

ME

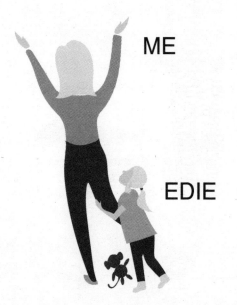

EDIE

WINSTON

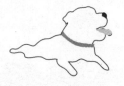

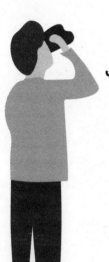

JOSH

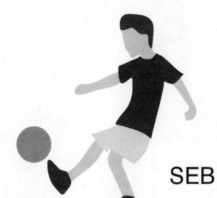

SEB

ISAAC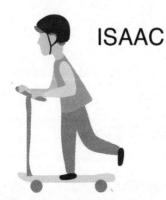

TALLULAH

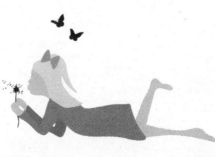

A quick note before you dive in.
If you follow me (*Part-Time Working Mummy/PTWM*)
on Facebook or Instagram, you'll already know what
I'm about. Feel free to skip ahead.

If you haven't ever heard of me before, I've included
one of my most loved posts from Facebook below to
show a little of what I do online . . .

The Mothercare Post

Today I popped into Mothercare – for no other reason than
my bladder is not what it used to be and it's the only shop
left in the world where you don't have a panic attack for
taking a piss for free.

As I was getting back in my car to leave, I saw a lady who
was struggling to get her pram out of her boot. I could see
she was on the verge of just reversing over it – meanwhile
her baby was having one of the best newborn meltdowns
I've ever heard.

Do I do what everyone else in the carpark is doing and pretend I can't see her and drive off – or do I try and help her? I decided to try and help. This 23-year-old beautiful girl was having a massive, 'What the fuck have I done?' moment . . . she'd stormed out on her boyfriend because he hurled the word 'depressed' at her in an argument. She decided to show him that he could go fuck himself and clean the house that he keeps moaning isn't tidy enough. So, off she went with her eight-week-old baby boy, only to drive off and realise she had forgotten nappies and spare clothes. Her baby had then done a thunder shit through his vest and his Babygro, which was now on the car seat. He was desperate for a feed and, because of his screams, her boobs were leaking through her bra, so she had driven straight to Mothercare, because somehow the thought of buying him new clothes and breast pads for herself, then trying to change this shit-covered baby and clean down a car seat while he was screaming with starvation in front of a shop full of people, was better than going home and feeling even more of a failure to her partner.

I got it. I got every single bit of it.

I remember Betsy arriving when I was 22 and turning my whole world on its head.

I remember feeling like I was failing every single day. I remember never experiencing anger like it at everyone but her, for being asked why I hadn't managed to run the hoover round, or when my mum started moaning about my dog being full of germs and getting too close to her, or my mother-in-law for asking why her cradle cap hadn't cleared itself up yet – everyone always assumes you're 'just coping' and cannot fathom out why, when they ask you what they deem to be a 'simple question', it sends you over the edge.

Then there are all the helpful diagnoses that everyone starts throwing about amongst themselves that they think you can't hear from the next room – that you've got 'a bit of PND' and you need to see a doctor.

Anyway, back to today – so I marched into Mothercare and bought breast pads, nappies and a vest, then went back out to the car and we nailed sorting the baby together – we scraped the shit out of the car seat with wipes (it's amazing how many of life's problems can be solved with a wet wipe). We then sat in the front seats of her car and she latched her baby on to feed while we chatted about how fucking hard it is to be a mum and how much our partners can be utter wankers at times and we giggled about how a human of that size can produce so much shit.

It became clear to me this girl just needs more love and support from everyone around her.

She needs to be able to sit on her bathroom floor and sob so much she's hyperventilating about how she's ruined her whole life, then half an hour later when she is crying with laughter at *Gavin & Stacey*, she needs her partner not to ask if she thinks she could be bipolar.

Her family need to listen to her break down about the fact she feels like broken glass is slicing her nipples off every time she latches the baby on to feed – she feels like she has no life as he has been stuck to her tit for the past two months since he came out of her fanny, which is also now ruined for life. They do NOT need to offer to go to Sainsbury's and buy her a box of SMA because they think it's clear 'breastfeeding isn't for her'.

When her partner walks in from work and sees last night's dishes still piled in the sink, it isn't an ideal time for him to mutter the words, 'What's for dinner?' Instead he needs to just wash up and tidy round, then offer her some food; this newborn 7-lb bundle of joy she's birthed has taken every bit of her energy today – she hasn't even had time to make herself a cup of tea, let alone turn into Nigella at dinner time, and he needs to not be a dick and meet the lads on Saturday night. Yes, it would be fun to go and get shit-faced, but there are plenty more Saturday nights for the rest of his life. I get she is an absolute cow to be around 99 per cent of the time but her whole body has gone to shit, her life is now controlled by another tiny human, and she doesn't have the choice to get dressed up and go and get smashed with her mates, so watching you getting ready for a night out is going to make this shit situation a whole lot shittier.

There's every chance she's going to lose her mind if her mother-in-law arrives one more time and comments on the fact the baby always seems to have that dummy stuck in his mouth, which HER son never needed. Right now she doesn't give a shit if he's sucking on that dummy at his 18th birthday party. She hasn't had a shower for six weeks without getting shampoo in her eye because she's having to sing 'Baa Baa Black Sheep' to this child who's screaming again for absolutely no reason whatsoever while he's wedged beside her in his rocker in between the toilet and the sink because she can't cope with the 'mum guilt' if she's in another room.

At the end of our chat I said to her that this is all so temporary. One minute you're at the doctor's being dramatic because your six-month-old has a rash on her neck, then what feels like five minutes later, you're back screaming for antidepressants because the same child didn't get her primary school placement and if she attends the school the council have given her, you've convinced yourself she'll be running the streets with a gun and robbing grannies by the age of ten. Then you get to where I am now, following my almost-teenager around in my car and checking her school bag and phone – praying never to find what I'm looking for, although I don't even know what that is.

So yeah, we worked out together that it's hard, whether your baby is thirty minutes old or thirty years, they are your baby for life – and once they come into this world everything changes. Forever. But at each stage, where you feel that you will never get through is temporary, so don't let it break you.

So that's just one of the posts from the blog I started two years ago . . . a blog that makes people constantly ask questions. Questions that no matter how many times I answer, more people join the page and ask the same question again . . .

So I decided to write a book to help you see the rest of the stuff that goes with it. The stuff that will make you say, 'Shit, I thought all these mummy bloggers just fucked about drinking coffee and writing a few posts on what shoes they bought this week while competing over who has the worst-behaved kid or who consumed the most wine. Because that isn't me, and that isn't *Part-Time Working Mummy*. The *PTWM* blog, the *PTWM* page, has some of the most amazing warriors you will ever meet. Their stories, their lives, break me every day. But I know them – I know them because they are me, and I hope I am them. I've been through it all and, while I still can't believe anyone is listening, I'm going to run with it while I can, because there are more women (and men, and teenagers) out there who need it, who need to hear that things will get better, that they are doing brilliantly, and that someone knows what they are going through. So, here we go – this is where this mummy blogger came from . . .

INTRODUCTION

It was 26 January 2016 and I'd had a twat of a day. I'd been angry, sad, upset and hormonal – added with a touch of parental guilt for a complete laugh, and my life had been turned upside-down about a hundred times since break-fast. As I threw myself down on the sofa waiting for the inevitable shouts of 'Muuuuuuuum' from my tiny turds – who would no doubt now be the thirstiest, hungriest, hottest or most unloved children who just needed me to give them food, drink or a cuddle instead of just going to sleep and allowing me to just sit, alone and in peace for an hour before I went to bed – I thought about something I had done earlier and wondered if it had been the right choice. On the way to work every day for the past ten years I had passed a woman on the local bridge, taking her kids to school, walking with her dog, having the time to do all the little bits that, as a working mummy, I never seemed to do. I'd watched her for so long, and when I got into work that day, I poured out everything I was thinking onto a local Facebook page.

Every morning for the past 10 years I've driven from Torquay over the Shaldon bridge on my way to work . . . and most days I've driven past a beautiful lady with crazy blonde curly hair. She started out ten years ago walking her eldest child to the primary school with her younger ones carried on her chest and in double buggies (she had a double buggy, one strapped to her chest in a carrier and two walking with her – five in total I think), while walking a beautiful retriever puppy.

Every morning I would watch her and be in awe of how organised she was, how she could possibly manage, and how happy her babies looked. I would then continue the rest of my journey to work with a lump in my throat that someone else was doing all of those things because I felt I should be at work.

This lady made me realise that, actually, I should work a little less, and learn to manage a little more.

So, as I drove past you this morning and saw you kissing your daughter on the forehead who I used to see as a tiny baby and is now a little lady, with your dog walking alongside at a much slower pace now he's so much older, and I imagine all your other children are now at secondary school and walk there by themselves, I just wanted to post on here, in the hope that somehow it will reach you, to say thank you; because of you I have now reduced my working hours so I can spend some mornings at home and doing the crazy school runs with all my kids. I make sure I go and fight back tears watching all their school plays and I bake (mainly inedible) cakes for the fetes, and I love all of it!

It's amazing that seeing a thirty-second glimpse of someone else's life once a day can make yours so much more enjoyable xx

---

I never thought for a second anyone would even bother to read it.

I never thought for a second it would change my life.

But it did. I sat there with my partner Josh beside me – giggling away at my forays into public posting – and I checked the post. I'd wondered if it might have got a few 'likes' or if anyone had commented something negative.

'Shit, Josh,' I said, looking at it and trying to actually compute how many likes there were, how many comments had been written, 'this thing . . . this post I did? It's gone absolutely mental.'

The words on that page changed everything when the post went viral. Within two days, I was contacted by pretty much every British newspaper. I had reached media as far afield as the USA and China, and I had *Good Morning Britain* and *This Morning* in a bidding war over who could persuade me more than the other to appear on their sofa and talk about the post.

It had gone crazy, and as much as I was in shock, it was a good crazy because I had written a post about someone that I was in awe of and who had touched my life, even though she had no idea who I was or what effect she'd had on me. Someone who was just another normal mum whom I had spent the past ten years watching doing the school run while I was on my way to work. Someone I needed to thank, and someone who had made me want to be a better mummy and change the way I did things. I couldn't believe it but there it was – the little bit of thanks I had given, the little bit of kindness I had shown in the post, had made people want to spread it all over the world. They shared their own stories, they tagged people who had made a difference to their lives, and they repeatedly wrote in the comments asking the writer of that anonymous post to begin their own blog.

So, I began searching Facebook for mums similar to me. I spent days on the Internet researching blogs and their content just to see what writing about your life involved, what reactions you got, and what people said to you and about you. I could find nothing. The only mums who did blog seemed to be nice, happy ones with their lives to-gether. They had a husband, a few kids, a mortgage, and a couple of nice cars on the drive. They had an annual holiday abroad and they lived lovely, simple lives. It was all picture-perfect and it was nothing like the life I lived or the life lived by most of the women I knew.

I had gone through life making mistake after mistake. I'd had a shitty childhood, got into drugs in my teenage years, and had had three daughters from two failed relationships. I'd been in an abusive relationship, been through loss and heartache, but I was still standing – and I felt that there must be thousands of women, just like me, who didn't have the Instagram dream, but who did need a bit of support to let them know that, actually, they were doing just fine.

So, I sat with Josh, my fiancé, who had brought another two beautiful kids into our full-time brood, and explained my dilemma – that the things I had to say were a bit different to any other Mummy Blogger. Would anybody want to hear the truth about what life was like as a mum and stepmum of five with a chaotic patchwork family? He looked at me and reminded me that there are more people in the world who make mistakes than who have their lives together. I might be one of the former, but there was a whole army of us out there.

And that was it.

Right then I decided to start my blog page, where I would talk honestly about it all. That night, *Part-Time Working Mummy* was born and I don't think I've paused for breath ever since.

This book is the next step for me. It's everything I've been through that's made me who I am, plus all the lessons I've learned along the way. I hope it will give you a bit of a laugh as well as the strength to keep going when times get tough. Because the reality is, we are all in this together . . .

1

ONCE UPON A TIME

I have very few memories of being with my mum as a child, but the ones I remember are so clear – right down to the clothing I wore, what fruit was in the brown bowl on the glass coffee table, whether it was sunny or raining, whether it was day or night. They're like snapshots that I can reach into and feel or smell; they're as real to me as sitting here now, typing this. I guess that's what we all wonder as Mommas – what will our children remember about us, about their childhoods? When we look around at all the other women who seem so perfect to us when we feel like crap, we assume that they are getting it right and that their kids will look back on the gingerbread houses they made together or the six-hour cupcake-making sessions, whereas ours will recall nothing but us shrieking 'Shit!' a hundred times a day while we search frantically for the car keys and scream at them that the dishwasher doesn't load its bloody self.

It's all somewhere in the middle though. We all have good days and bad days, and the bad days make us feel like the good ones don't happen that often. So, despite everything about my childhood and the million questions I could ask my mum, I remember good times. I remember snoozing with her on the sofa in the afternoons while my elder siblings were at school. She would lie behind me and spoon me into her, and we would nap together while my favourite film, *Annie*, played repeatedly on the TV in the background. I remember her smell. To this day, I could still pick her sweet perfume on her warm skin out of a thousand other smells.

When I was little, my parents had moved from Denton in Manchester and bought a country B&B in a little village in Devon. I think they made this choice to give us a better life; maybe keeping track of us in a rural setting seemed like it would be an easier task. But it turned out we weren't the picture-perfect family, and I picked up on that before I could even work out specifically what was wrong in my parents' relationship.

I remember Mum being sat surrounded by Dad's paperwork in one of our many upstairs bedrooms. She would be on her knees with piles of invoices and receipts around her, and she looked so sad. Now, as a parent and a grown woman, I see that look with more clarity: she was trapped, desperately unhappy with little support.

It seemed to me as if she and my dad were constantly arguing, the sound of their fights coming through from the kitchen below my bedroom as I lay on the floor and waited for them to stop. They never seemed to, as it just went on and on and on. I never remember being scared of either of them – they were both good, kind parents. The shouting didn't seem aggressive, just emotional – and incredibly repetitive on my dad's part. I would often go downstairs to ask for a drink in the hope it would end their fights, but I'd just be handed a bottle of juice and have to toddle back to my room, where I would lie on my floor again and listen to their rows continue.

Our house was crazy. Nowadays mine is too, but, growing up, it was different. The house was always full of people all the time – family and friends from Manchester, but maybe they felt that because our home was a B&B, it was fine to just land there and stay for a while, certainly most weekends. My siblings always had their friends over too.

There are fond memories, too, of course. I clearly remember our milk lady, a woman called Sue, who would come round every morning and deliver the glass bottles of milk for us all – she had really long dark hair that would always be in a high pony tail and she would open the front door calling 'Wooohooo'. We also had a 'Video Man' who would rock up every Friday night, open his car boot in the street, and show everyone the hundreds of videos he had for rent. I would get a *Care Bears* one every week and one of my brothers would get a *Star Wars* one.

What I remember, above anything else, is how loved I was. I remember that feeling of being such a loved child; I was shown affection constantly and I knew that my mum just adored me so very much. One thing that does stick in my mind was that she lived for interior design and gardening – she would spend hours at her sewing machine making matching lampshades, bedspreads and curtains out of Laura Ashley fabric, and our gardens were like something out of the Chelsea Flower Show. She would host the most amazing parties where people would turn household items into musical instruments and dance until the early hours of the morning; there would always be so much amazing food with full cooked breakfasts, three-course lunches, homemade sweets and cakes, tables groaning with the weight of it all. It was a happy home in that respect. My Aunt Marg and Mum's friend Hazel always told me they envied Mum because we had it so right as a family, together, all of us.

But it couldn't have been right – not really.

I don't remember her ever saying 'goodbye', I don't even recall how or why she left, whether there was an argument beforehand and she left in temper, or if she just slipped away in the night. I was certainly never told anything by anyone at the time, but one day I woke up and she just wasn't there anymore.

I know the date. I know that Mum moved out of the family home on 16th January 1986. I was four years old, with my siblings ranging in age from nine to eighteen.

On Valentine's Day, as I remember it – a month later – one of our neighbours moved in with her two kids. She was our neighbour, but now she was also my dad's girlfriend. As a young child, you accept what goes on around you because there is trust in the adults raising you. You think that, no matter how hard it feels, what they do and say is right and normal; you ignore that ache in your heart and you think that other children live just the same as you do. It's only when you reach a certain age that you look back and see that so much of that time was never, ever right.

My dad was always a workaholic, he never hid that and it was part of our world; he always said it was so we could have the nice things in life. He certainly continued to work even after Mum left, and that was hard because he was often far away from home and it meant that we were now pretty much solely raised by his girlfriend, our new 'stepmum', Pamela.

Pam was the opposite of my mum in every possible way. I had spent my first four years with a woman who adored me, who despised bad language, and who rarely raised her voice. My new life was very different to this. I never remember feeling anxiety until then, yet now it was with me day and night, sat in the pit of my tummy, whirring away like a physical illness. I don't want to go into the details because what matters is how I came through it all, but the things I went through certainly had the effect of making me want to rebel as a teenager. It's only through extensive therapy as an adult that I've learned about ways in which people can control behaviour emotionally as much through threats and implication as physically.

In the middle of it all, Mum would phone me and my siblings. I don't remember much in terms of how often she called or how much we saw her once she had left. My memories of that time are not really there. During therapy sessions as an adult it was explained to me that, as a child, I wouldn't have been able to cope with all of the feelings that came about from my mum leaving, all of the heartache. Which is why as an adult I don't have those memories because your body suppresses them in order to protect you. I do know that she first moved to a house nearby with her new boyfriend and I know from there they moved to Birmingham, and I know from there they moved to Lincolnshire. Again, I don't remember lengths of times or dates but I remember her feeling so very far away from such a young age and with the distance (which was now a seven-hour car journey away) came the reality that I now could only see her a few times a year. I don't know what made her make those choices, as a mum myself. It's not something I will ever be able to make sense of because I miss my children when I'm at work, which is a twenty-minute drive away. But Mum still always continued to phone. During those phone calls, I would be sat in the hallway upstairs, and, strangely, I recall every detail – we had a mushroom-coloured house phone with a big round dial. It sat on a wicker shelf but the phone wire was long enough that you could stretch it and sit on the bottom step. I would use my finger to try and wipe the dust out of the round holes where the numbers were or wrap the curly cord round my wrist while tears ran off my chin. I had to learn very quickly not to cry. I suspected that Pam was listening out downstairs in the kitchen because, any time I did begin to get upset, I remember she would race up the stairs, grab the phone off me and slam it down, while screaming things about my mum.

I would then be given the option to stop crying immediately or go to bed. I always chose bed, as my heart hurt too much to try and force my tears to stop falling. A lot of the time when I climbed into my bottom bunk it was still so light outside, bright sunshine blazing through my curtains, but I would just cry myself to sleep into my pillow. I had no idea if and when I would speak to or see my mum again and I worried that she thought that I had put down the phone on her. As a five-year-old girl, these responsibilities weighed heavy on my mind. When I look back at that scene now, I can see the whole image, even down to the clothes I had on and the white bedspread decorated with pink clouds that I was laid sobbing under.

I cannot feel the pain but I can recognise how shattered my heart was; I can picture myself struggling to catch a breath because I am crying so hard. When I look at me as that little girl, consumed with grief at losing her mummy, the confusion and hurt I was trying to deal with makes me wonder if any amount of therapy can ever get you through such utter heartbreak. I believe that sometimes when something hurts you so much, it stops hurting at all.

The only respite I got from my home life was when I went to my best friend Leila's house. Leila had two older brothers, one of whom, Jamie, was best friends with my brother Matthew. Leila's mum, Sammy, was the kindest, calmest, most loving lady I have ever come across in this lifetime. Every time we saw her she showed Matthew and me the love we desperately craved. It was the same love our mum had given us, the love a mother shows where they genuinely want to know what you've eaten at school, if you've had a good day, how you are. The love where they remind you to drink your juice so you don't get dehydrated. The love where they force you into that bath you desperately don't want to have because it's nice to smell clean. You don't forget that sort of love when you're going through hell. I am still in touch with Sammy today and I spent New Year's Eve 2018 with her and her family. As we sat in her beautiful home, I thanked her for all she had done. I told her that I didn't feel like I have it right like she did, because there are times when I lose my shit with my kids, I get annoyed and I don't hold it together and all I ever remember is her holding it together. She responded by saying, 'You know, Rachaele, as long as your kids know how much you love them when they fall asleep at night and when they open their eyes in the morning, they'll be fine. The rest of it is just personality'. Sammy is proud of all I have achieved. I think she knows more than anyone that I almost took a different path, so she sends me a text every now and then reminding me that she's proud, or that she loves me, or that she's always there if and when I need her.

Leila lived in an amazing bungalow which seemed absolutely huge when I was little. It had windows the whole way round and you could run round the outside of the entire house in a circle. I often go back to that house now. I park up and just look at it. I don't know why. It's almost like some kind of therapy, although now it looks so tiny. In my head, it was always the dream house that I would buy for my own family one day because of the memories it gave me, but the reality is that my army would never fit in it, so instead I occasionally drive past. I pull up and walk past on the pavement, I check if the hole in the bush that we used to run through is still visible, I note the changes – like all the fruit trees that sit in the garden now full of apples and pears which were once open spaces where we played bat and ball or put up a tent to sleep under the stars, and I feel thankful, because, once upon a time, that house and the family that lived in it were my saviours.

That lovely home sat a five-minute walk away from Broadsands beach. Broadsands is a big beach, it goes on and on with golden sand and has the prettiest pastel-coloured huts all along the front and, in the summer, there would always be hundreds of people behind wind-breakers eating sandwiches out of big plastic cool boxes. The bungalow was surrounded by fields where we made dens in the woods out of black bags and anything we could take out of Leila's dad's shed (if we were confident he wouldn't miss it!). Matthew and I were happy there, it was like having a little piece of our childhood back, even if we only had each other rather than the rest of the family too.

Sammy let us stay over whenever we were allowed, she never said 'no' to us, not ever. She took us on their family holidays, even to Fuerteventura for a fortnight on my eleventh birthday. By now, my dad had no idea where I was as he wasn't hardly around. Pam must have been happy as she didn't have to deal with me if I was somewhere else, so as much as I could, I'd be at Sammy's house.

My eldest brother and sister had left home pretty much instantly after Mum disappeared. They couldn't deal with the changes at home.

During these years, I had no idea where they moved to.

I don't recall ever seeing them other than every Sunday morning at 10 am when John would come and take me out for the day. This was the only day of the week I would wake up with a different feeling in my tummy, a nice butterfly feeling rather than fear or apprehension. We would race round in John's B-reg white Vauxhall Astra then go to the house of his girlfriend's parents. Della's mum and dad made us Sunday roast and, while John and Della spent the afternoon cuddled up watching the Grand Prix after the food, Della would let me go into her bedroom and play. I would dress up in her expensive clothes and shoes, putting on her lipstick, playing the Beverley Craven song 'Promise Me' over and over on repeat! I would rewind the tape to the beginning time after time, and sing it to my mum like she could hear me, feeling like my heart was breaking.

John and I would then sit at the dining table and write our mum letters and cards. I would draw her pictures which John would post to her in secret without Dad and Pam knowing anything about it. I knew from the start that things like that needed to be kept a secret from my dad and stepmum, as did the phone call I made every Sunday afternoon from Della's dining room.

John would then announce it was time for me to go home and the anxiety would hit my chest like I'd been winded. The good butterflies would leave and the nasty ones returned – and the tears would come. John would make me so many false promises about how things would get better, and about how Matthew and I would soon be back with Mum. I never saw it then, but when I picture his face now, I can see his heart was also broken with the heavy responsibility he had to carry as he tried to protect his baby siblings.

So that's where I began . . . and I'm conscious that my childhood wasn't all rosy, but I wonder how many people can truly say they had an amazing childhood. So many of us go through things as children that were never what they should have been and I want that out there – I want people to understand things aren't always perfect.

And ultimately you learn, no matter what kind of childhood you have, you learn . . . and here's some of what I learned from those years:

- You never know what's round the corner, so make the most of the good stuff while you can. When you're a kid, you can't really think that way, but even if you have been massively fucked up in childhood, try to hold on to any little things that can make you smile. I think of how much Mum loved me when she was a mum to me, the music filling the house, the food she made, the affection she showed – so now I try my hardest to make those memories for my children while they grow.

26

- Try to recognise that we're all muddling through. When I say John made false promises, I don't mean that in a bad way; I mean that he couldn't control the behaviour of the adults in our lives, so he did what he could, and he always loved me. He wasn't lying, he was just trying to make it easier for me to go home. Give people credit for what they can do, not what they can't.

- There are decent people out there – Sammy and her family were a godsend to me. That lady was a good mum and a good person and I learned so much from her. Listen to your kids, pay attention to the small bits of their lives, and if you are able to, love their friends because sometimes it changes lives.

2

A FAMILY
FALLING APART

Matthew took Mum leaving the worst, I think, and I
often felt a rage come over me when I saw how he was
treated at home and the lack of support my father gave
him – it was as if no one seemed to get just how much
he had been affected. I loved my big brother so much.
Even though he was older than me and bigger than me,
I still wanted to protect him. I hated anyone who hurt
my brother and I believe both my father and stepmum
should have seen that he was crying out to be helped
through this confusing, horrible part of his life that he
never asked for or deserved to endure. I suppose to Dad,
every time he came home from working away, he was
having to hear how badly behaved his two children had
been while Pam's got glowing reports. He probably felt
sorry for her having to look after us. Things worsened for
Matt – he lost his way for a little while. He left home as
soon as he was legally allowed and we lost touch for a little

while as my world continued in the same pattern. John always told me that Dad had promised he would never marry Pam. I don't know why that was so important to us all back then, as children – but I suppose marriage seems so final and forever. While they remained unmarried we lived in some hope that him telling her to leave was likely to happen

All of that was really my life, for ten whole years. That feeling of anxiety now lived inside my tummy, day and night. Every night when I got into bed I prayed to a God I no longer believed in to let me dream of 'My Little Pony' cartoons and seeing my mum. I made a secret vow to myself that when I grew up, I would love everyone's children, no matter who they were.

My mum still lived in Lincolnshire, which was a 12-hour coach journey that I now made with a friend twice a year. I was around 12 years old at this point. Mum came down during other holidays, but I think seeing her almost made it harder for me to cope without her. She was still the same mum. She seemed so maternal when I was with her. She still smothered me with love and affection, and her Mancunian accent was still as strong every time I saw her and she was nice. She was never nasty about my stepmum or Dad. She didn't speak badly of them or say horrible things and I remember that. But she also never explained anything . . . and still to this day I have never had an explanation, not really. It's something, as a family, we haven't ever talked about. Not with Mum or Dad, not as siblings together, it's just something we've accepted happened. But if I am honest, especially more so since I have become a mum myself, it has left me with so many unanswered questions and unresolved issues in my mind. That's why I now try to explain situations as much as I can to my kids. I have to accept now that I don't know if any explanation would ever give me enough justification to accept her leaving us, and moving so far away knowing we desperately wanted her, needed her. So sometimes I feel like the elephant is still in the room and other times I feel like it's something I want to pretend never happened.

Still, my mum felt like home.

A home I no longer had.

Mum would say her goodbyes at Leila's house due to not being welcomed by my dad and stepmum. What started out as me being a little girl sobbing into Sammy's arms on the pavement while waving Mum off when she drove away, turned into me being an angry pre-teen trying to chase the car while being restrained on the roadside because my heartache had turned to rage.

By the time I hit my teenage years I rebelled. I wanted out of that house and away from Pam – and I was willing to do anything for that to happen. I knew I needed to fight. I would have to be independent . . . But when the reality hit and I got my wish, I didn't follow in her footsteps quite as well. At this stage, Pam was losing the little control over me she had left. Dad was still working away as hard as ever, and I felt like I didn't know him anymore. He only knew me through what she told him, so we were further apart than ever. I was just the 'problem child' he returned to at weekends and he did nothing more than discipline me. As much as the worry around my stepmother was still inside me, it was quickly being replaced with an anger I had never experienced before.

I continued to get into trouble at school so I confided in my form tutor, Mrs Jones. Mrs Jones was a really firm teacher; she took no shit but I felt that, deep down, she quite liked me. I was so frightened about telling her what it was like at home, but it ended up being the best decision I could have made. She was my lifeline.

I can't remember the exact words I used, but I could tell Mrs Jones didn't know whether to believe me or not. By this point I was heading off the rails at school. I had been caught truanting and she could probably see I was heading for a bad place. What I was saying must have been awful to hear as a teacher, but it was her job to protect me and she did just that.

Children's Services were called in for a meeting at very short notice; along with my dad, my eldest brother John, who was now 29, my Head of Year and me. I remember Dad started the meeting blaming anyone but himself or Pam. He told them I was out of control and impossible to live with. I had got involved with older boys by this stage and had started drinking alcohol, so he hoped people would believe him as there was that 'evidence'. He claimed that Mum was at fault because she had left me ten years earlier, he claimed that John was at fault because he shouldn't be getting himself involved. He stated he had worked hard to provide for his family and he believed my stepmum could not have raised us any better. He continued through the meeting trying to blame everyone except himself – although, actually, a lot of what he said was true. I was now drinking alcohol at weekends, I was getting involved with boys older than me, and I was probably not being a very nice teenager, but I felt that he didn't want to help me, but that he hated the embarrassment of having to sit in this meeting.

I remember John staying silent throughout, but repeatedly shaking his head every time our dad made another invalid point. I think he was probably in both shock and disbelief at my dad's take on the way he had seen things. John had been raised by both of our parents for the first eighteen years of his life. I think in some ways it must have been harder for him to have witnessed what Dad had let home become for us after, once upon a time, being a good father.

Children's Services gave immediate consent to me being removed from my family home to live with John under an Interim Care Order. It felt like a lottery win.

John drove me back home the next day to collect my

belongings. I remember skipping into that house full of confidence because I was convinced that things were finally changing. For years, I had gone through mental and emotional suffering, but now I felt that I was free of it all. I went up to my bedroom and all of my belongings had been placed into two black bags. Pam was nowhere to be seen. As I walked out of the house, Dad was waiting at the top of the steps in the driveway. He had the same look upon his face as he did after Mum had gone; he looked broken. He was trying to stop himself from crying and he asked me not to leave, but it wasn't his choice any more. I didn't answer him; I just carried on walking down the path. I had my whole life in those two bags and I remember feeling nothing but utter disgust at the situation we were now in.

I think I lasted about six months at John's. At the time, he lived in a one-bedroom flat with his girlfriend and, as amazing as they both were, they had their own issues. My behaviour was getting worse, and John just didn't have the time to manage me while trying to set up his own building business. It was also costly – he lived in a different town to my school so he was having to fork out for bus fares and lunch money, buy my clothes and shoes, and give me pocket money. John got no financial support for caring for me, which made it tough.

I don't blame him at all for what happened next – we decided together that I would go into foster care. I guess you always want your 'real' family more than anything else but sometimes that just can't be. John, without doubt, has always been my hero and remains with that role today. He was almost fourteen when I was born and I love him to bits. However, I am one of those weird people who, for some strange reason, pictures my life after the people I love have died. I read about a child abduction or murder and I put myself there, physically, as that mother. I don't know why I do that because it makes me feel the most horrific things and have the most appalling thoughts. It makes me so emotional, but maybe this is what makes me want to help others. So, every time I see John and I leave him, I do the 'What would I do if he died?' question, and it frightens me. It genuinely terrifies me. I imagine the same way a daughter would feel about a loved father dying, because it's the same relationship. It's a need, because every time I have ever needed anything I have gone to John and he has never let me down. Over the years, I have massively fucked up, but I call him and he sorts it out for me without question.

John has such a calm, rational head. I have never seen him get angry, not once. And always as I was growing up, his words remained with me: 'Honesty is the best policy; no matter how bad it is, lying will only make it worse.' He is fun, he is happy, he is chilled out and he made a choice not to have children because, I believe, he felt it was his job to raise my brother Matthew and me.

He made a commitment to himself that he would always prioritise us. Even now, when the shit hits the fan and I call him, he is there making everything OK. He talks sense – and he makes all the time in the world to sit and talk that sense to me. He explains why I feel the things I do, why I behave in the ways I do, and he keeps me calm when I am in a state of panic. I have never known John to fall out with anyone. He refuses to get drawn into feuds and he has a way of pointing out people's wrongs and rights without ever being nasty, rude or cruel.

Matthew is different – he is complicated, and I believe this is totally down to his lost childhood. I do believe that when our family was destroyed, he was broken in some ways and I have cried many tears over that; he's my brother, no matter what, but there is something about having a childhood that changes so much that one day everyone is envious of what you have, the next day a stray dog wouldn't want it. That has to have some lifelong effect on you. Matthew has two children of his own now, and despite splitting up with their mum eight years ago, he understands that I stay in contact with her and that I love her. Sometimes they fight and fall out and sometimes they both call me and rant, but he knows I will not get drawn into it because she is a good mum. She wants what's best for my niece and nephew and despite the relationship between her and Matthew, she has never stood in the way of allowing me, their paternal aunt, the type of relationship my children and I have with them, which is an amazing one. Deep down, she also just wants her children to have a good childhood where they are loved and prioritised by both their parents. I cannot ever ask for more than that. Matthew is the best storyteller and he makes my tummy hurt every time I see him because he is so funny. He is the sibling I call on my way to work when I'm bored because he will always make me giggle and when he's having a bad time, even when that's brought on by his own decisions and actions, my heart still aches for him because when you go through something together, so closely like we did, there is an everlasting bond there that only you understand, together.

They were both always there, giving me love when I needed it, although in different ways and at different times. Looking back, I can see things much more clearly, but, back then, I had no idea that a time was coming when my own self-destructive behaviour, which had been fuelled by what had happened to me as a child, would be heading towards a horrendous point.

I was fifteen at the point I went into foster care; I was placed with a family closer to my school and my first foster mum was actually an amazing woman. Mary was a single mum who idolised both of her daughters, and it is testament to my time there that one of those daughters remains a best friend of mine to this day.

Mary worked hard to provide for us but, because of

this, she was out of the house a lot, meaning that I did as I pleased. I started missing school again and hanging around with other children with similar issues to mine. I wasn't being the easiest child in the world and Mary had her own family to deal with. A few months after I got there, Mary's eldest daughter became pregnant. It was a difficult time and we were sharing a single room, so I had to leave to make space for the baby.

I moved foster homes and lived with a lady called Debbie, her husband and four daughters. Debbie was a Brummie who lived for her kids. Her house was chaotic, but it was full of love and I felt like it was a real home for me at last. Her daughter Hayley and I were inseparable. They had no money really – it was my first experience of living on the breadline and it taught me an important lesson. When I lived at my dad's, we were reasonably wealthy; although he didn't spend much money, we had a huge home, we ate good food, we shopped at Sainsbury's, and I grew up knowing that cash was never a worry and it was something that until I had lived at Debbie's I had definitely taken for grant-ed; money was never something that I saw Dad and Pam struggle with or even discuss. When I moved into Debbie's, I saw that, for some, money was extremely tight and it was an eye-opener. When something was gone, it was gone. If something like shower gel or toothpaste ran out, that was it – there was no cash to simply get more that day, or to go to a well-stocked cupboard where there were spares. We ate dinners like egg and chips on a regular basis because they didn't have the money to feed us all meat, but what I learned from it all was that it didn't matter. Debbie was a million times happier than my stepmum, she was nicer, she was loving and her home was a lovely place to be. Her door was always open to all of her children's friends, no matter how troubled they were. She never judged, she just loved and listened and advised anyone as best she could and I remember thinking she was the type of mum I wanted to be when I had children. Even though she struggled to pay her bills, she still made it a priority to sit me down and ask, 'Rach, are you OK?' She adored her family unit despite her financial struggles and the strain upon them, and it was the first time I realised that money isn't something you need to be happy in life.

By now though, I had totally lost my way. I was going out every weekend taking illegal drugs. The rave scene was massive back then and there was a club called Plymouth Warehouse that we would all drive down to at about 10 pm every Friday night. We would wear luminous lycra spaghetti tops so we glowed in the UV light, and we'd spend the whole night dancing. I had lost all my school friends due to truanting and began hanging around with much older people who were a really bad influence on me. I was taking ecstasy, acid and whizz on a regular basis at the club, and, after it shut, we would go back to some-one's flat or house and carry on for hours. I would then bunk off school during the day. My life was spiralling out of control.

I knew I had to make a choice.

Before I had left home I had babysat for a lady called Suki who had split up from her husband. She was in her late twenties and had a little girl who was four. She used to let me stay over on a Friday with my friends and we would go to a club called face 2 face, which was an un-derage disco. In return, on the Saturday night I would babysit for her daughter so she could go out with her friends. Although they were all around fifteen years older than me they all looked out for me, so I decided to give her a call. I explained how bad things were and she im-mediately offered me a room in her house. By now I had one black bag of life belongings which I packed up and kissed my amazing foster mum goodbye. I promised I would remain in touch with her because she had been so good to me. I left Brixham that afternoon. By now, I had dropped out of school, so that wasn't an issue. I'd sat a few exams but I didn't really have a clue what I was doing because I was either coming down off a drug binge or gearing up for the next one. Right then things were at their worst. I knew it was make or break. I needed more, I wanted more. I didn't want this disgusting dirty life I was living, I didn't want the reputation I was quickly gaining and I didn't want to be the next teenager to die of a drug overdose.

●

I'm always honest with readers of the *PTWM* page and I'm being very honest here too. You might be wondering if you could be drinking a bottle of wine rather than read about my problematic childhood, but hopefully you'll see that I'm doing it for a reason. I think that we have to focus on the shit bits and not bury them away because if we do that, we don't allow them to change us as people, and sometimes the shit bits can transform us into amazing beings that are far better because we have learned and we have grown differently. I think we can understand each other better if we know where we've come from.

● When I was in foster care, I learned a lot – maybe not then, or not all of it then, but certainly there are things I look back on, like people opening their homes to me out of kindness when they didn't have to. That has shaped the person I am today, so when Betsy introduces me to one of her friends who I can see is a bit troubled, I don't advise her to end the friendship, I don't make them unwelcome in my home. I let them in and I love them and I hope that, as an adult, they will look back and remember our home and the people in it as the family that always cared and made things a little bit better.

- Debbie and her family possessed very little, but they had love. Debbie was richer than Pam would ever be, and she made me feel loved in a way that no overflowing cupboards or non-stop supply of toiletries ever could. Your kids will remember if you're a Debbie, truly they will, so don't worry if you can't afford the limited-edition Nike Air trainers every other child is rocking around in because when they look back on their childhoods, what they will remember is who gave them love and time. That is more important than any material gift.

- I've never forgotten what John always told me – it's a cliché, but he's right: honesty is the best policy, and lying will only tangle you up in knots and make things harder. You need a good memory and a lot of energy to be a good liar, and I've been there, I have told lies at some points in my life and it's a huge regret, it's something I have definitely learned from. Now, no matter what the situation is or how bad it feels, I hope my children know that things will always work out better if they are honest.

3

MISS INDEPENDENT

After moving to Torquay, which was two towns and a forty-minute bus ride away from where I had grown up in Brixham, I wanted to believe I was far enough away to not ever go back.

I thought I could change things if I worked. So, I did – I worked hard, day and night. At the same time, my school friends were collecting their GCSE results and choosing colleges to begin their careers with support from their parents, but I was applying for jobs alone to be able to pay my rent. I got my first job as an administrative assistant at a local newspaper and worked there nine to five during the week. I then got a second job in a hotel, where I waitressed six to nine every evening, as well as weekend mornings. I really wanted to ensure that I had no time to party, take drugs, or make any more mistakes.

I was working at least 70 hours a week and, other than paying my rent and food, Suki banked the rest so that

I had some savings behind me. It wasn't long before I decided that I was sorted and I wanted to have my own space. I found a bedsit in a little place in Torquay, which consisted of a tiny bedroom with a cooker and sink in the corner, a lounge with a sliding door and, behind that, a shower, bath and toilet. I remember I couldn't afford an ironing board so John came round and made me a board made out of plywood that would sit over the cooker, I would place a towel on top and have a makeshift ironing board. I look back now and have a giggle at that, as it must have been the most dangerous ironing board in the world!

The bedsit was in an old Victorian building. The carpets were burgundy with a busy gold print all over them and the high walls were woodchip painted in magnolia. It was incredibly dated but clean. I felt proud of my little flat. I had a single bed, a sofa and a wardrobe; there would be nothing else for a while until I had saved up, but what I did have was all mine. I used to sit in my bed late at night after finishing work, marking the yellow plastic kitchen accessories in the Argos catalogue that I would save up to buy. Here I was, a sixteen-year-old fighting hard and being Little Miss Independent. Living in this flat also gave me the first taste of a few things that have informed my adult life. However, it was when living here that I had my first experience of domestic abuse, and the effects it has on children. In the flat upstairs lived a couple with five children. He worked full-time and she was a stay-at-home mum – and he battered the shit out of her whenever he could.

He would mostly beat her at night, but his temper was fierce at all times and I would hear him run across the floor so that my ceiling vibrated when he was in a rage. It sounded like thunder. I would lie in my bed, petrified, listening either to screams from the kids or cold silence. I have never, to this day, worked out which was worse.

When he was at work, I would often go up and see her. There were seven of them crammed into a tiny flat. She would be covered in bruises and she would cry while her kids clung to her arms and legs, fighting each other to get as close as they could, just to hold her. I wonder now if it was their way of making her feel safe, or them wanting to feel safe, or maybe a bit of both.

'He's a good man,' she would tell me. 'A good husband, a good father.'

'Then why does he do it?' I'd ask.

'He's stressed, he has a stressful job – and he gets so tired, and upset . . .'

Her excuses for him were just that – excuses (and I've seen and heard them plenty since those days), but I just couldn't understand. I begged her to see sense. I would offer to stay with them and call the police but she refused. Over time, the attacks became more frequent, the mixture of screaming and silence became more regular, and the bruises became a deeper shade of purple until one day I went up there and she was crying for a different reason – because he had left her. He had been having an affair with a colleague at work and moved out. She was broken-hearted and, although she couldn't see it, I knew it was the start of a new life for her and her children. I had no idea that she would be the first of many such women I would meet in my life, or that the issue would become such an important one to me.

Soon after moving into the flat I met a boy called Martin. We were the same age, but he was much taller than me and he had his brown hair styled in 'curtains', which he grew long enough to tuck behind his ears. He had cute freckles on his nose and the biggest set of perfect white teeth I'd ever seen. He always dressed well and smelled amazing; despite him only being sixteen he was always in designer clothes and I liked him *so* much. I really, really liked him. Martin had no worries, he was just fun, all the time, a real cheeky chap. He was laid-back, kind, and just made me happy, made me laugh and he made all the things that felt bad and crap in my life disappear.

My bedsit was a few doors up from the hotel that his parents owned. He had four older siblings, and the whole family had moved down from London where they had run markets. They were all proper Cockneys, an extremely close-knit bunch, and fiercely protective of Martin. His grandad was one of the nicest, most genuine men I have ever met and I still remember all the amazing stories that I would sit and listen to for hours and hours, although it took me ages to understand all his Cockney slang.

I still felt unhappy underneath though and I suppose I started using drugs as an escape route at that time. Martin hated drugs with a passion back then but he loved me. He really loved me. His parents didn't seem keen on our relationship because of who I was and what they perceived me to be. From very early on they put rules in place which made us being together so hard. I suppose looking back on it now as a mother I can see why they might have made those decisions. They were trying to protect their son from a young girl who was extremely damaged and although I think I understood that, I also craved to be a part of their family unit because it was something I had never had. And now, as a mother, because of my childhood I can't help but look at it the other way round because of who I am. Love can heal many things, and if any of my children ever grow up to choose a similar partner to what I was back then, I would approach the situation so differently because of who I am now, and I can't help but wonder, if they'd taken me in and loved me as one of their own, things may have ended differently.

I continued to work but I hated the newspaper job so I wrote letters to all the local dental practices – it was my childhood dream to work at a dentist! I practically begged all the practices in Torquay for a position as a trainee nurse, and, as I hand-delivered all the letters, I told the receptionists on the desks that I was available to start immediately and I would take a crap wage!

One surgery replied to me the following week and invited me in for an interview on a sunny Friday afternoon. I remember sitting with the dentist. He chain-smoked continually throughout our interview in his surgery and asked me lots of questions. I remember instantly feeling at ease as it was more of a chat than an interview and the questions he asked were about me, who I was and what I did, the reasons I lived alone and not with my family – it was never about why I wanted to work as a dental nurse or for him. He showed a genuine interest in my life in a friendly way – he just seemed curious. It was clear that, as a father, he struggled to understand why I didn't live with my mum or dad. I remember feeling quite privileged that he paid an interest in me as a person. He offered me the job and I started at 9 am the following Monday. I would be paid a trainee wage of £80 per week. That Friday felt like it was the best day of my life.

But when I look back, dental nursing was definitely my first experience of how women can be bitchy with one another too. I had to quickly learn how to fit in though, and be the one who slagged off the girl who had just walked out of the staff room. What was at first unsettling very quickly became normality, but it was a normality I was never comfortable with. It's strange how negativity is often a default behaviour for people – and it's sometimes hard to see that it doesn't have to be like that.

To add to the challenge of living independently at sixteen, working for £80 a week and having a troubled relationship, I was also caring for my nan at this time. She had been taken to hospital with pneumonia. My nan had three daughters – my mum and her two sisters – but they all lived hours away, and other than visits from her grandchildren, she had no life at all. She refused to socialise and would sit in her flat day and night, occasionally walking to the local shops but other than that she would chain-smoke Lambert & Butler cigarettes, watch the snooker and do *Take a Break* crosswords. I loved my nana; she was like my mum, kind and warm. She had Estée Lauder lipsticks that I would smear across my lips that had a beautiful smell to them that they no longer seem to make these days. She used to make me salads in a bowl and she would lay perfect pieces of hard-boiled egg on top that she had cut with her egg chopper.

When she was poorly, me and my cousin Samantha were really the only ones that visited her each day. I think everyone was so used to Nan always complaining she was old and unwell that they didn't think it was serious and so no-one visited her more than normal. As teenagers and young adults everyone becomes so busy with their own lives that they never really stop to think about the day that person isn't around anymore. Mum and my aunties didn't come down and at the time I was 17 and getting a lift to the hospital every night after work from the hygienist who I worked with at the dental practice, a lovely woman from Stoke-on-Trent. When I got to Nan's ward, she would tell me she had spilt more tea on her nighties and underwear, which I knew was urine because it was now more and more clear she was worsening and was now becoming incontinent. I would sit and do crosswords and spoonfeed her her tea. I would hold a carton of Ribena to her lips so she could drink. I would deliver her freshly washed clothes each evening and take away her dirty ones, promising her I would wash off the tea and return them the next day. I would then catch the bus home and get everything sorted for the following evening. I would buy her *Take a Break* each week.

This became my routine until one day I arrived and Nana had worsened, badly. The only way I can describe the noise she made was like a wheeze so bad it sounded like a rattle, and she had no idea who I was. At that point I lost it. I went to the nurses' station and told them she was dying. I started shouting, asking if the reason they were leaving her to rot from pneumonia was because she was 82 years old and they couldn't be bothered to give her the care she clearly needed . . . They asked me to calm down and as I waited I overheard one of the nurses saying to Nana, 'Ethel, this is unfair, you need to be honest and tell her.' I remember that feeling of my heart breaking. It was a physical ache and the lump in my throat grew so big and painful I couldn't swallow it away. I remember going home to call my mum and when she answered I anger-cried. I shouted that her mother was dying and her and her sisters needed to be there. By the end of that call I was on my knees sobbing. I had cared for Nana for what felt like forever and I probably knew how unwell she was, but actually, the realization that she definitely wasn't ever going to get better hit me and I just didn't know how to cope. Also I think the responsibility I had just hit me and I felt like I had failed her in some way because she wasn't going to survive much longer.

The next day after work I arrived at the hospital and my brother Matt was in the waiting room outside the ward. I went to go in and he told me we weren't allowed. I walked in but was ushered back out by my uncle, my auntie's husband. He told me Nana was in a bad way and it wasn't good that I should see her like that. I remember feeling so angry, beyond angry. I wanted to scream 'Listen you, I have been here day and night doing this shit for months, I've seen her at her fucking worst when I've been washing her piss-ridden clothes that no-one else has cared about – most of which I have with me now clean and I need to get her changed and give her some fresh Ribena and this week's magazine.' But I didn't, I accepted her children had now arrived to care for her. I sat in the waiting room and waited to be called through by them.

When I went in I realised my uncle was right: my nana was dying. She was in her final stages and it was a sight I could never have prepared myself for and one I can still picture to this day. I was broken. So were her daughters and so were my siblings and my cousin Sam. I imagine Mum got that call from me and thought I was being my usual dramatic self, but she and her sisters drove down anyway and I don't think any of them were prepared for the sight that met them: their beautiful momma in the final stages of lung cancer, having kept it a secret from everyone because she didn't want to 'upset' or 'bother' us. It was my first experience of 'good lies', when someone keeps something from you, or lies to you because they haven't got the heart to break yours. I went in and sat at my nan's bedside for hours. As I got up to leave, with all my family behind me, I leant forward and kissed her forehead. Her skin was still as soft and silky as ever and as I said goodbye, she reached for the Ribena and pointed to her lips. I gave her a drink, then she kept signalling for me to leave the Ribena closer so she could reach it because she thought she was being left on her own. My sister began to cry and said, 'She thinks no-one is here. She thinks she is by herself. She thinks we are all leaving her.' I tried to explain Mum was there but she was in and out of consciousness and had no idea what was happening. That image still haunts me, and as I write this I cry, because cancer really is one of the worst ways to die, no matter what your age.

My mum and her sisters sat round her bed all night. The following morning they left her to get breakfast quickly and when they got to the canteen my nana passed away. They say you choose when to go and I honestly believe that. My nana didn't want any of us to suffer at her suffering, ever.

My nana is the only person I've loved, properly loved, that I have lost to death. I suppose given the fact I am now 36 and I have met and loved so many people, you could say I am quite lucky, but on that day, 8th April 2000, I felt like the unluckiest girl in the world to lose someone I loved so much. After she died and my heart was shattered some more, I was about to hit self-destruct all over again . . .

●

Looking back, I can see that the pressures in my life were building. However, when you're young and trying to break free it's hard to recognise the signs of things getting too much. If I could speak to my sixteen-year-old self I would tell her:

- I'm proud of you.

- Hold on to your independence and your ability to look after yourself, hold on to the sense of care and the love that you have for people that cared for you.

- Remember to take care of yourself, you're going to need it.

4

TOXIC TIMES

So, that was going on behind the scenes of my new independent life. Nothing is ever simple, right? I stayed in dental nursing for eighteen months. I enjoyed the job, I adored the dentist I worked for, I loved my patients, but I simply could not live off the wage any longer. My rent was now £60 per week and I was still working almost 80 hours between two jobs just to pay bills, bus fares and food. I couldn't afford to buy clothes or shoes, I couldn't learn to drive. The reality of being an independent teenager was smacking me straight in the face, so I began to look for better-paid jobs.

Quite quickly I found a new job in 2002 – a care support worker for young adults with autism and Asperger's Syndrome who were sectioned under the Mental Health Act. The pay, to me, was amazing and rather than clear £600 a month for working 77 hours a week, I was now getting £1400 for working just under 40 hours. Luckily,

I loved the job too. It was challenging but it was fun. I really liked caring for others and knowing I was helping to give them a better life. The staff team was diverse, with older nurses and younger carers, but it worked well and we got on like one big family. I felt like I belonged there. Through earning much more money than I was used to, I was able to buy nice clothes and to start having nights out again – but with that came alcohol and drugs once more. By now, cocaine had hit the nightclubs and it was so easy to get hold of, anyone who was anyone was doing it. My weeks soon consisted of going out clubbing Thursday, Friday, Saturday and Sunday nights, then spending Monday, Tuesday and Wednesday recovering with a come-down and hangover. Looking back at that situation now really devastates me because I was so lost, and the thought of one of my girls ending up like that makes me feel physically sick, but I suppose that's what makes us the parents we are because of the life experiences we endure.

My amazing wages were disappearing fast and my amazing relationship with Martin was going to shit. I treated Martin really badly towards the end of our time together. I was 19, still young, but definitely old enough to know better. He had cared for me for three whole years, had been nothing but a gentleman and had showed me how my life could have been, but I just kept on fucking it up. I was trapped in a cycle of destructive behaviour and

I couldn't get out. He begged me not to take drugs and I'd be on the phone to him promising I wouldn't, while I was going out to meet another dealer.

I would ignore his calls at 2 am when he would be sat outside the nightclub in his car waiting to pick me up because I knew it would be the end of us if he saw my drug-fuelled state. However, it was never enough to stop me. It's difficult to explain now why I kept doing what I was doing. But there eventually came a time when Martin just couldn't do it any more, and because of the hurt I felt at my own behaviour, I just kept getting worse. I flirted with other guys in clubs and I trampled on Martin's heart even more when I knew I had already broken it. I remember my heart breaking a little bit too. I was broken that I could be so horrid to someone who had done nothing but love me through some of the most difficult years of my life. I begged him to take me back and promised I would change, but he knew I wouldn't and, deep down, so did I. Shortly after we split up, he left the area to move back to London, and I had no choice but to try and heal without him. Now, it's clear I needed to make some changes to my life when Martin left – only it wasn't so clear to me back then. I moved into a flat-share with my friend Stacey, because I couldn't bear my own company – I was drowning in loneliness. Through therapy I have come to realise this is due to the fear and devastation of abandonment from my childhood, and although back then I gave Martin no choice but to abandon me, when he did I just stopped coping. I thought a change of scene in a new flat with my best friend, rather than a change within myself, would help. I've now learned that while it might feel like you want to just run away, you never really start to feel better until you confront the difficult things and understand yourself.

●

Stacey had grown up travelling all over the country with her mum Helena. Helena was amazing to me from the minute I met her. She never judged, she could see all my faults, but she just loved me and welcomed me because she had made mistakes in life too. I really loved her in return. Stacey and Helena had a role-reversal relationship whereby Stacey was the sensible, hard worker, and Helena just wanted to party and have fun, even though she was the mother – but it worked, and they idolised each other.

Stacey and I lived in a flat above a garage, rented to us by my sister's husband. The flat was bare and, as much as we wanted to make it a home, we never had the funds or the time to do much to it, so we lived in each other's bedrooms and pretended that the lounge, kitchen and bathroom didn't exist. We would eat beans on toast or pasta and cheese most nights and watch TV together in her bed. I remember always feeling safe with Stacey; she was like my big sister – always looking out for me as no-one messed with her – not in a bad way like she was a frightening person, but because she was one of the kindest, most selfless souls I have ever come across. I suppose growing up like she did made her have no fear about taking any shit or standing up to anyone. I liked this feeling of being protected, but I hadn't yet worked out any of my own problems properly.

I was still reeling from my broken relationship and I was still going out a lot. I was a regular at a local pub managed by a real womaniser called Tony. He was almost ten years older than me, but always showed an interest, offering to take me and Stacey home after we'd been out for the evening. So many people warned me not to get involved – especially Stacey – and I always promised I wouldn't. He was old (or he seemed old to the teenage me), he was a cheat, and he had three young children. His relationship with the mother of his daughters was very much on and off, and everyone knew she led a dog's life because of him; he made it no secret that he cheated on her. Tony started coming round at night after he finished work, bringing us food from the garage and just watching TV and chilling with us, but then he began buying me gifts. They were the sort of gifts I could never buy myself because of the price and, within two weeks of the presents starting, he had ended his relationship – for good, he claimed. He then arrived at my door with all his belongings.

It all happened so fast and I didn't know how to handle it. I felt a tug of war going on around me. Stacey told me that, if he was moving in, she was moving out and I remember feeling suffocated from the very start. This wasn't what I'd wanted: I needed my girlfriends around me to help me heal from Martin, I didn't want or need a relationship, especially a complicated one where children and ex-girlfriends were involved, but he was relentless – it was as if he had decided on a campaign to get me no matter what I said. I would arrive home from work every day and continue to be showered with expensive gifts – on top of that, he began telling me he loved me, he would leave me voicemails on my mobile where he was playing love songs down the phone, and I almost felt owned. Looking back, the only way I can describe it is it was as if I had been bought and I now belonged to him. I didn't have the strength to distance myself back then. It's so difficult when someone bears down on your space, your emotions and your time. You can quickly become overwhelmed. It gets even worse when that person is volatile, and also when you haven't been raised around positive love it's so easy to mistake negative as good.

One weekend, three weeks after Tony had moved in, I knew that Martin was down from London, as one of our friends had told me, so I went out to the local nightclub to try and see him. He ignored me most of the night but, as we still had so many mutual friends, we all left the club at the same time. He was walking ahead of me with Stacey and some others when Tony pulled up and got out of a car that didn't belong to him. He later told me he had borrowed it in the hope of following me to 'catch me out' without me recognising him. He mounted the pavement, then jumped out and ran over towards Martin, instantly head-butting him. I saw Martin knocked unconscious and lying on the pavement; he didn't even see it coming in order to be able to defend himself. Tony was going crazy, screaming and shouting and foaming at the mouth, he looked deranged and the group of us, about fifteen in total, just looked on in utter shock and disbelief. Tony then dragged me into his car in front of everyone. I can honestly say I have never, ever, felt fear like it. I actually urinated myself as he was driving while he was screaming at me that we were going to Berry Head to kill ourselves together off the cliff edge. As we sped through town, I just wanted to die there and then. I didn't want to die with him though, so I opened the car door as he was driving and jumped out into the road. I remember bouncing like a ball down the road until I was knocked unconscious.

When I came round I was on the pavement next to Tony's car. I was informed by the ambulance driver he had been arrested at the scene and was now in custody – he told me his car would be towed away. I looked like I had been in a car crash and I felt like death; amazingly

I had no broken bones. I was told I was lucky as I had jumped out at a taxi rank where cars were slow moving or I could have died. The realisation of the type of relationship I was in had hit me and I felt so, so frightened. I called Stacey who was at her mum's with Martin, so I got a taxi there. I walked in and couldn't believe the state Martin was in – he had two huge black eyes, and my feeling of self-hate for what he had endured because of me came flooding back. He had barely even looked at me all night and he still ended up black and blue.

I had a shower and put some of Stacey's clothes on, then we sat with Martin and Helena in the lounge talking about everything. It was like a debriefing after a trauma incident. I felt so physically sick my tummy hurt and I had a lump of sadness in my throat for what I had caused. Martin stayed with me that night and cuddled me to sleep; if I'm being honest, I would have cut my own arm off at that point for him to have taken me back. I missed him like I had once missed my mum and my nana, but I knew I had caused too much damage and even getting on my knees and begging him wouldn't have worked.

The next morning, he left for London, as he was running a successful business by now; he had moved on and was coping without me. I remember his words before he left: 'Always remember your worth,' he told me, 'don't ever just settle, Rach.' Those words have always stuck with me, mainly because I forgot them so many times over the years, but also because I know I hurt him and yet he was one of the good guys, and we shouldn't ever hurt the good guys.

●

This part of my life was such a whirlwind. It would be a while before all of these events sank in, but I've now learned a lot from them and can see how I wasn't in a good place. When you are in the middle of lots of drama, it's difficult to pinpoint the exact things that are making you behave in a certain way. People under stress and going through difficult times can act irrationally, and I understand that now – although I didn't analyse much at the time. When I look back, I can see everything more clearly and I often think about how it's all impacted me in later life. From now on, I'd also like Martin's words in neon lights in front of every woman in the land as she goes about life: 'always remember your worth'. We should never, ever forget that.

● Try not to break a good guy's heart because, if you truly are a decent person, your heart in turn will break at the damage you cause. Be honest if you don't love them or, if it's not right, end it, but don't stay because they're too nice to let go of, then end up destroying things far more. Sometimes, no matter how nice or loving someone is, they're just not meant for you.

● Being bought gifts is nice at times, but remember: being bought a bunch of cheap roses by a lovely guy at the start of a relationship is by far a better feeling than being bought an expensive watch at the start of an abusive relationship. No matter how nice lavish gifts are, always watch out for the warning signs.

● Domestic abusers work hard. It's draining to keep a victim under control – abusers plan, they think ahead, and they are clever people despite society portraying them so very differently. Abusing someone to the point they still stay in a relationship with you takes a lot of time and effort. Remember this, look out for it, and educate your children because domestic violence within teenage relationships is devastatingly apparent.

5

A BRAVE FACE
AND A NEW BABY

After Martin left, I went back to the flat and got into bed, just wanting to hide from the world, but later that day Stacey answered the doorbell and in walked Tony's six-year-old daughter. Even though it was still early days into our relationship I had spent a lot of time with his daughters; I liked spending time with them. Now his eldest was at the door and said she wanted to tell me she was sorry for what her daddy had done and gave me a huge bouquet of flowers and a card from M&S, a card I have kept to this day, written by her and signed on behalf of her two younger siblings. I felt her visit was a warning to me from her mum, Tony's ex, that this is what life would become if I stayed but I already knew that I had made my choice – to be with Tony.

I made sure I wasn't in the house when Stacey moved out shortly after the incident with Martin, as I knew what I was doing shouldn't be happening and I couldn't face her. It wasn't what we had planned less than a year earlier and I knew I had massively let her down. I didn't see her much after she left, but then I didn't see any of my friends any more. They couldn't understand my choice to be with Tony and it was easier for me to hide myself away from them all. I continued to work hard and I became a stepmummy to Tony's daughters, aged six, two and one. They were gorgeous children and, when I was with them, they helped heal all my broken bits. Tony's ex-partner was left shattered by their split and trying to cope as a young mum on her own to such young children with minimal support was really hard for her. It also helps me to totally understand how so many women who have got out of an abusive relationship are still very much victims because the control never goes away; it's there just as much, if not worse, through the children, financial, or in whatever way the perpetrator can still find to be controlling, and this is the life the woman still leads, despite being apart from him. Once you've let someone in, it's hard to flush them out.

The girls were really the first children I had ever been round as an adult. I learned quickly how to change nappies, make bottles and read them stories as they drifted off to sleep. I was thrown into it all very quickly but I also loved them very quickly too. Tony continued to run pubs, so he was only home between 3 pm and 8 pm each day. He worked long hours at weekends and my only company was the girls and my work colleagues.

I need to jump forward a bit here, so bear with me because this part matters. Since I began *Part-Time Working Mummy*, I have learned about the cycle of domestic abuse. This cycle is real, it's there, but it's hard to see when you're in it and this is what happened to me, right from the start. The highs were amazing. We went on trips away, holidays, nights out. I was lavished with gifts, and I felt loved and protected. He was an amazing father so I had the family I had always dreamed of and I could pretend that all the bad stuff was over – until it started again . . . and it always did.

The lows were horrific. The violence was present from the start but over and above everything, it was the fear of being trapped. There are certainly incidents that have never left me, certain times I screamed at his eldest daughter to call the police while he screamed at her not to and she stood there, a rabbit in the headlights in total fear of who to listen to. It was devastating and it leaves me to this day filled with a feeling of guilt that makes me feel sick. One night there was an incident which was so bad people outside our flat heard.

Suddenly, I heard a banging on the door and, hoping I would be saved, I began screaming as loud and as hard as I could for help. Tony immediately left and, I guess, headed for his car. Minutes later my work colleague walked in and came up the stairs. He was friends with my neighbour, who had called him upon hearing my screams. I still remember his face when he saw me; there I was, fully clothed, sat in a bath of freezing water while my flat was trashed. He ordered me to get washed and dressed as he was driving me to the police station.

I was seen immediately as I had visible injuries.

I remember the officer who spoke to me. He was young, with dark hair and he was really nice, and he went out of his way to reassure me that if I gave a statement, Tony would be arrested. That terrified me. I thought of the girls, of the times he was nice, and I just couldn't bring myself to do it to him. It all seemed far too serious.

I left the station. I went home to grab some clothes and my colleague drove me to a Birmingham service station where my mum collected me and took me back to her flat in a sleepy little town in Lincolnshire. I wasn't having much contact with my mum around this time, but I would speak to her throughout the month and the contact we had was good and positive. I think the difference in what my mum saw of me since we saw each other six months earlier shocked her. My weight loss was horrendous – I was now skin and bone. My pelvic bone stuck out so much it felt sharp. My whole face was covered in spots and I lived with constant mouth ulcers that made it even more difficult to eat, but, more than that, I was no longer me. I had been replaced with someone I no longer recognised – but the appalling truth was, I was also someone who desperately missed the person who had turned me into this. That's the reality of abuse. And so, the following day, Tony arrived after making the eight-hour drive to Lincolnshire, with a huge bouquet of roses and drove me back home. Mum took me to one side and warned me Tony was bad news – but she knew I had made my mind up so she kissed me goodbye and as I left she was crying, and she whispered in my ear to stay safe. I hoped that, by leaving him and our home, I had shown him I wouldn't allow things to continue the way they were and that things would get better.

•

When you think of someone who is subjected to domestic abuse you see them as a victim, you see that they are always the one to get hurt and upset but, the truth is, at times in my relationship I was just as bad and I believe that's what kept me there. I look back at the venom I spat or the fights we had where I tore flesh. I bit, kicked, punched, hit, and it makes me feel sick that I could ever have behaved like that towards another human being. When you are in a relationship so toxic, where you are so controlled and so conditioned, sometimes you don't know how to react. There were moments when I got so angry at my situation I wanted to make him angry too so that he would lose his temper – because once he had and we had fought so badly he would feel as bad as I did. It could turn into some kind of gang war where we wouldn't stop until we were just exhausted, having kicked shit out of each other and said things that couldn't ever be taken back.

There were days when I hated myself so much for getting into this situation that I would purposely wind him up because I didn't want him sat there thinking things were OK while he was watching TV and I was running round after everyone yet again. I was genuinely exhausted. I was working full-time, doing everything at home and looking after all the girls while he would just sit, in front of the TV, ignoring us all and at times it would send me mad. I would purposely annoy him to the point he would lose it, sometimes with violence but sometimes he would do things back to me to make me turn as crazy. He would wait until I was asleep then put the bedroom light on and turn the TV up full blast. He would open the bedroom window in winter when it was freezing. He would wait until I had put the shampoo on my hair in the shower then pull the electric cord to cut the hot water off – I would come out fumbling and pull the cord, wait for the shower to heat back up and as soon as I got back in, he would pull the cord again. These sorts of behaviours were constant, they were repetitive and sometimes I felt like I was losing my mind, and, at times, I would. Sometimes I got so angry I would self-harm in front of him. I'd rip chunks of hair out or punch myself repeatedly in the head while screaming because I didn't know how to cope with the anger.

So, I stayed. And plenty of women do. You stay because you start believing it's your fault, that in some sick, twisted way you must enjoy a fucked-up relationship like this, and when you are told that you are as much to blame as he is, that you are totally to blame, you start to believe it.

There is a horrible predictability to what happened for so much of it, but it won't surprise anyone that the next stage of the relationship was when I became pregnant the following year. While I have never doubted my love for my firstborn baby Betsy for one second, it did come as a huge shock. I was so thin and so unwell that my periods were never regular, if they came at all, and I certainly wouldn't have been able to keep any contraceptive pill down because I was constantly sick after panic attacks or anxiety. I remember secretly doing the pregnancy test in the bathroom of the new house we had moved into. Not for a minute did I think it would be positive and, when those two blue lines appeared, I was violently sick with shock.

I continued being sick while muttering 'fuck' over and over again. I sat on the bathroom floor leaning against the bath panel in total disbelief and called my brother Matthew. I laugh at that now, that of all the people I could have called I chose him. I don't know why, because at this point in my life we rarely saw each other. He lived away in Bristol and contact between us was rare but I think I called him because I knew he wouldn't judge, he wouldn't be negative or nasty, and he wouldn't be disappointed in me, he would just take it for what it was. I knew out of anyone, anywhere, he would make me feel better about what was feeling like the worst situation of my entire life. I was right – he just pointed out the harsh, stark facts about how things would become if I chose to keep the baby. I discussed all of my options through big fat sobs and felt devastated that I'd allowed this to happen. My parting words to him were, 'I'm going to have a termination, Matt – and I'm not telling Tony.'

I sat there for a few moments, knowing the enormity of my decision but also feeling that I just couldn't bring an innocent child into this. I would love a baby, I had no doubt about it, but I could see the effect the situation was having on Tony's girls and I just couldn't let another child go through it. It would be a huge thing to keep this secret and to end the pregnancy, but I had to be strong.

I put the phone down and prepared to follow through on what I had decided.

I opened the bathroom door and he was there.

Tony was there.

He was in the hallway and he had been listening to the entire phone call.

The argument we had was horrific and it ended with me being told I was keeping the baby no matter what I fucking thought. I had been irresponsible enough to get pregnant and there was no way in this world that I was allowed to do anything else, he told me – no one was murdering his baby.

I spent the first few months of my pregnancy in total denial. If I'd informed my work I was pregnant I would have been taken off duty due to the challenging behaviours our service users displayed, so this was my excuse to keep it a secret from everyone, when actually I just couldn't bear to face everyone's disappointment and the reality of the situation.

My baby was due at the end of August 2004 and that summer was incredibly hot. We moved house again during my pregnancy and now lived above one of the pubs Tony was running. It was a beautiful flat but it was in the middle of town with no outside space, our bedroom sat over the DJ box and the noise was horrendous. I don't think I slept more than three hours a night for the last month of my pregnancy. I remember one afternoon a week before I was due, I was getting so hot that my body was swelling more by the hour. My toes and fingers were huge and I was now sweating so much I was dizzy. I walked down to my GP and saw my midwife, who ran some quick tests and informed me that I had pre-eclampsia.

I was rushed to Torbay Hospital accompanied by Leila (remember her?), her wonderful mum Sammy, my sister, and Tony. Back then, there were no restrictions on the number of people you could take into the labour ward with you, and they were all allowed to stay with me throughout.

My labour lasted 28 hours. I was in and out of sleep, I had every drug going, and I was absolutely exhausted. The nurses put yoga mats on the floor so my friends and family could also sleep and rest, but I was in agony. I tried to keep going but, in the end, had to have an epidural as I was struggling to cope and I was really worn out.

My baby girl arrived at 4.43 am weighing 7lb 7oz. She had a mass of black hair and immediately latched on to feed from me like a little piglet. I named her Betsy. I have heard many women say they didn't get that sudden rush of love, that they felt nothing when they saw their babies, and while every pregnancy and birth book in the land reassures us that this feeling is normal, for me it was the opposite. I knew instantly. It was the first time I had ever been in love, properly in love. The second I laid my eyes on her tiny body covered in blood and gunge, her little eyes struggling to open, and her tiny white fingers wrapped around mine, I knew that I would die or kill for her without question. I promised her, in a whisper into her perfect tiny ear, that I would never, ever let her down.

My Betsy.

My friends that had had children had warned me in every gory detail about labour and the aftermath. I am one of those weird people who needs to know it all, no matter how bad or scary it is. I had wanted to hear everything: the drugs, the pain, the afterbirth, the stitches, what pissing the first time felt like – the lot, and I don't believe they held back in telling me. I still wasn't prepared! About 9 am the morning after Betsy arrived, I was in immense pain down below. I kept lifting my nightie up for a look, and there was what looked like a blood-coloured tennis ball sat in between my legs. It was throbbing and I couldn't work out why none of them hadn't warned me about this part of the process. I kept mentioning it to the care assistants and they reassured me it was all part of the joys of afterbirth. The pain continued to worsen and the tennis ball turned into the size of a small melon. I started losing consciousness and another mum on the ward noticed the blood all over my bedsheets so shouted for the nurses.

Within what felt like seconds my bed was surrounded by doctors and nurses. I was in and out of sleep while hearing them talk about emergency surgery, blood transfusions, and trying to locate my next of kin to sign some form. I don't remember feeling scared by this point; I don't remember even thinking of Betsy lying next to me in her plastic cot. I just remember feeling like I needed to sleep and I couldn't physically stay awake for a moment longer.

I woke up hours later to be told I'd had a vulval hae-
matoma. I had been taken to theatre where the doctors
had performed emergency surgery to cut it, drain it and
stitch it up. I then had blood transfusions and a catheter
fitted. I was then stitched front to back. The pain was still
horrendous. I was told something about an internal tear
being missed but I wasn't sure of the ins and outs – I just
knew I would be staying in hospital for the next few days
to recover.

Most of my friends visited over those days, even my old
best friend, Hannah, which surprised me. Hannah and I
went to school together but we weren't particularly close
then, she was in the year above me and was stunning,
the most popular girl in school who everyone wanted to
know. We had also worked together at the dental surgery
for a while, and became inseparable. I also loved Hannah's mum, Helen, a woman who worked so hard; she
had a beautiful little home and she lived for her children.
There was another reason I loved Hannah – she had an
older brother called Josh who was just as gorgeous as her.
He was quiet and shy but he had made my heart beat
faster every time I saw him because of how ridiculously beautiful he was. When I first became a dental nurse
I was really close to Hannah and during the week we
would stay at her house. She lived there with her mum
and her brother; her dad had passed away the previous
year and it was clear all three of them were trying to live

with a broken heart. Helen invited me into their family immediately and she would make me dinner every night and breakfasts before we left for work in the mornings. She doted on her children despite losing her husband, her soulmate, in such a cruel way. At the weekends we would stay at my house in Torquay; this was where the clubs were and we would spend the weekend going out together. We were never apart.

When I got together with Tony, Hannah was livid. She was really angry that he was so much older than me; she was aware of his reputation and she saw the massive change in me from being a partying hard, fun, outgoing girl to a stepmother of three young children who never left the house other than to go to work. She grew tired of arguing with me about me leaving him but eventually accepted my choice and things did stay amicable. Hannah came to the hospital to meet Betsy, but I knew that she, like all of my other visitors, felt the visits were tinged with sadness at what I had become and the life I was leading.

Unsurprisingly, I suffered with postnatal depression. Immediately. I arrived home from hospital and my dog excitedly jumped on the bed to greet me, but there was a feeling to being back that I couldn't shift. Mum had arrived down to see me from Lincolnshire and would be staying for a few weeks to settle me in – I was glad of that but there was a downside too. My mum is an amazing 'sorter'. She can tidy and potter for hours and make any house into a home, she enjoys ironing and cleaning and she loves to look after people. Anyway, she started shouting at the dog – he couldn't be near Betsy because he was full of germs, he would lick her face, or, worse still, if he landed on her with his weight and size he would kill her. I knew Mum was only trying to protect everyone, she was trying to help and part of what she was saying was right, but the anger that brewed inside me wasn't normal. He was my fucking dog – he was the only one who loved me all day every day, even when I was a shit owner who hadn't walked him; even when he had been to the vets and had had an injection, he always loved me and if he wanted to jump on the bed to meet Betsy he should be able to be allowed on the fucking bed.

Instead I didn't shout back, I didn't react. I just cried silent tears on my own in the bedroom that no-one saw.

The feeling of unhappiness, desperation, loneliness and an awful empty feeling consumed me. To this day I cannot explain it. I just felt so, so sad all of the time. Sad and angry, raging and desperate – and I could never explain why – all while trying to put on a brave face.

I felt I was the only mum in the world who struggled; I felt I was the only one that had these dark thoughts. I felt a shitload of guilt at having them and not being like everyone who seemed to thrive on motherhood, who seemed to cope, who seemed to enjoy getting up at 3 am to feed a baby or change nappies. So, I hid my feelings. I pretended I was just like them and enjoying every minute of motherhood.

Breastfeeding almost killed me. On reflection I think it was so hard because there isn't enough awareness about how much it fucking hurts! It is a pain like no other. Like other women, I was used to having my breasts touched, and I would often check them for lumps, but having them sucked and grabbed all day every day is not something my breasts are used to coping with. If someone had warned me about the sheer agony I was about to endure, I would have coped far better. Yes, I probably would have still sat on the edge of my bed with a pillow in my mouth to bite when she latched on. I probably still would have begged and pleaded with every member of my family to go to Boots and buy me tubs of formula because that tiny mouth of hers clamped around my nipple was causing me more pain than she ever did when she came out of me. But I would have been prepared.

Now, I warn women everywhere. Any pregnant woman or new mum who is breastfeeding, I tell them the truth – it fucking wrecks. No-one ever tells you but, believe me, it's like shattered glass slicing into your nipples. Until your boobs get to grips with the change that they are now udders to keep a tiny human alive, it will be hell. Get shares in Lansinoh, smother it on even when you think you don't need to, and have a pillow ready to bite down on when they latch on. Two weeks, give it two weeks, and after that it will be like a walk in the park, I promise. People have thanked me for that advice, because without it they say they would have given up, and I always said it needs highlighting more – a book on 'The Pain of Breast-feeding' should probably be my next one! If you don't want to go through the pain or you find it's all just too much, then bottle-feed, who cares? Your body has now gone to absolute ruin thanks to this bundle of joy, so as long as you're keeping it alive with milk, I truly believe it doesn't matter which sort.

In spite of my mum's advice, the dog loved Betsy, as did her three elder sisters who helped me bathe her, put her to bed, and helped wind her after I fed her. What was getting worse right now was my relationship with Tony. He still ran the pubs which meant that he would be gone by 9 am every morning to take a delivery, he would then pop home for a few hours in the afternoon but, because he was tired, he would sleep, or lie around irritating me while watching TV. He would then go back to work again and return anywhere between midnight and 3 am. We still lived above the pub at this time, and he had come up with the genius plan of having topless barmaids to make the business boom. The CCTV was rigged up to our flat upstairs so that he could keep an eye on things when he wasn't in the pub; but all those twelve cameras did was fuel my paranoia and make me sink deeper into depression, watching him cavort with the young, petite, beautiful half-naked girls behind the bar with their pert tits out on display.

I remember Christmas Eve 2004 so very clearly. Betsy was four months old and I had my three stepdaughters overnight. Tony was working downstairs, the pub was heaving, and the barmaids were, again, topless. I watched him chatting to two young blonde girls. He then walked over to the bar with them and clicked his fingers to the barmaid to get drinks for them all. They continued to chat and laugh as he handed them free drinks then he slowly pushed their heads together so they began kissing each other. He then put his head in between them and I saw the three of them tonguing and caressing each other.

I thought I was going to vomit. I was like a maniac, sat there breastfeeding my baby in the dark while studying the CCTV of my partner full-on tonguing two other women while his three other daughters were sleeping in the room next to me. I settled Betsy in her Moses basket and started running down the stairs towards the pub. I had fake-tanned that night to make myself feel a bit better for Christmas Day. The only fake tan back then was St Tropez, which needed to be left on for 12 hours; when you applied it, there was a green tinge all over that made you look like you were starting to rot. It also smelled rancid. So here I was, a bright green psychopath, sporting a headband to keep my greasy locks out of my face, while dressed in a milk-stained dressing gown, sprinting down the stairs ready to lose my mind, but as I got to the bottom step, he opened the front door.

The row that took place that night was one of the worst. It was extremely violent, while four babies slept above us waiting for Santa to come. Christmas Day was horrific; I was battered and bruised while pretending to my family that everything was fine.

It was a mask I got used to wearing.

⬤

When I pack this part of my life into a chapter like this, it does seem that an unbearable amount happened: gaining a family, being thrust into being a new mum to an unplanned baby, dealing with mental health issues and domestic violence. But even during this time, when I was a desperately unhappy shell of a person, there were still rays of light. There were still times I was happy and grateful for things that I had. I found out who my true friends were – and my amazing daughter came into my life.

⬤ I chose to cover the breastfeeding because, for me, and so many other women I now speak to, it's the one 'bad' memory that's always remained with us. The debate between breast and bottle is out there so much and the debate can be fierce, but I refuse to participate in it. Many amazing adults were fed formula and they turned out just fine. Do what you need to to keep well, because, ultimately, if you are killing yourself to please society, your baby isn't getting the best from its mama.

- My postnatal depression stands out here, but so does the domestic abuse – and these two together are a killer, mainly because so many women I now work with have been left paralysed with fear that they will have their children taken away if they leave their abusive relationship while they're struggling with postnatal depression. It's a favourite for perpetrators to tell their partners and one that I hear daily. It's also bullshit. You don't lose your baby because you are unwell – you will be given tools and support to cope, I promise.

- And if you have a friend who is in an abusive relationship? Just be there for her. Supporting someone suffering from domestic abuse is, at times, one of the most frustrating things to do. You might not understand why she doesn't 'just' leave. But if you read up on the cycle of abuse, you might. It's not as easy as just packing your bags and heading out. Be patient, please be patient, because she needs you. She needs friends and she needs not to be judged. There will hopefully come a time when she decides to go, and that's when you can swing into action – but, until then, just support, just let her know that you care without making her feel shit about something else she hasn't managed to do.

6

BROKEN HEARTED

There were other changes in my life too, not just Betsy. Tony encouraged me to have a relationship with my dad because he hadn't known his real father and he hated his stepdad so he used to play the 'What if he died?' card, which made me feel like a shit daughter. It was something else to be added to the list of how crap I was.

I saw my dad away from his house for the first few years, away from my stepmum. He would come and cook for me on a Saturday afternoon as that was one of the things he loved to do. My favourite meal is liver and onions but I cannot for the life of me cook it. Every week he would show me how to roll the liver in flour then fry with onions and make the tastiest gravy, so I looked forward to him coming over and, I suppose, looking after me – like a father should look after his child. And he did, he did it so well. He was also amazing with the four girls and he would tell them stories about what he got up to when he was young. He would play games like 'chopping off his thumb' or putting his fingers through flames of fire, and they would watch in amazement and he would make us all laugh until we cried, because, when he is happy, my dad one of the funniest, kindest men I have ever been around.

I was in my early twenties by this point and it was the first time I really felt like I knew my father. He still worked hard, and far away from home. Pam didn't seem particularly close to her own family and as much as I never wanted to feel happy at someone's sadness, I did. I believed she had her karma, sat in a huge, once-beautiful home, all alone. I started going to the house with Tony and the children, just for an hour on weekends at the start. Pam was there and, as far as I was concerned, she hadn't changed. It seemed clear to me that we shouldn't make ourselves at home, whereas her grandchildren from her biological children had their own bedrooms in that house, full of toys that our children felt they could not touch. I knew I would always try to make no difference between Betsy and Tony's girls as long as we were together as I've always believed that children shouldn't pay the price for the behaviour of adults.

I don't know if Dad saw how she was and chose to ignore it, or whether he just wanted a quiet life and chose to pretend it wasn't happening, but I believe he knew. He wasn't stupid and the way he acted when she was around was totally different to how he was when she wasn't there.

I had that same feeling of anxiety in my stomach when I was around her and now it seemed that it was there for my girls too, I couldn't bear for them to ask her anything. Children that are raised with love are naturally curious, they will touch things, say they want a drink, moan that they are hungry. They want to explore but being there filled me with the same sick, anxious feeling I grew up with.

I tried to see Dad as often as possible away from his house and I always made out to him that I was lucky to have met Tony and that I was happy. He knew how much I loved Tony's girls and I think I always wanted to prove to him that I did OK on my own, without him. I think deep down he was really proud of me and I think he believed that I was happy.

By this time, I was still working for the same company but had moved up the ladder and held a demanding position within the senior management team, I had a new company car and earned a good wage. My house was a home, I cooked and cleaned, and I knew all this made Dad proud. He always 'secretly' gave me money. He would shove a wad of notes into my pockets and say, 'It's between us.' I always protested, even though most of the time I was drowning in debt, but he wouldn't take 'No' for an answer. I think it was guilt money actually; guilt because he had let me down massively and he would never really be able to make it up to me like he should. I felt like I had a dad though, and my girls had a grandad. Although he had no idea how unhappy, trapped and desperate I was, I knew that, if I needed him, he was there, at the end of the phone. By now we spoke every morning when I drove to work and most evenings he would call me from his van. He still worked away and despite getting an allowance to stay overnight in hotels he had a mattress in the back of his van where he slept. He would shower in the services where the lorries park and he would go into a supermarket late at night to get reduced food. He would make me laugh until I cried by telling me he had bought a roast chicken for a quid and some out-of-date rolls which he would use all week for breakfast, lunch and dinner. It felt good to have him back. Until one day, Pam announced that they were getting married. I couldn't believe it – after all these years, how could he do what we believed he would never do? How could he marry this woman?

I left for work on the Monday morning after I found out, and my heartache turned to rage. I had a shit day and got home late. I put the girls to bed, then Tony and I began fighting. I can't remember what it was over but it escalated quickly and he lost his temper. He knew he had gone too far so, as he left for his evening shift at work, he locked the front door behind him so I couldn't escape. The back door was open but we had built the gate up to over six foot outside and it was kept locked and strengthened because our dog was amazing at absconding. I was now trapped in the house, but it was a regular thing and it didn't bother me. Half an hour later the doorbell rang. I opened the letterbox and it was my dad. I told him Tony had accidentally taken the key so I couldn't let him in. I knew he thought I was lying so I told him to climb the gate if he wanted to come in – and he did. The sight was so funny – and, as shit as the situation was, it still makes me giggle to this day: an overweight 50-year-old man with a mass of ginger hair scaling a six-foot-high gate while muttering swear words, attempting to break into his daughter's house to speak to her! By the time he walked in the lounge he was seething.

'What's going on?' he demanded.

I wanted to let my rage out so I don't think I left a thing out of what it was like at home for me and my siblings while he was away grafting to give us a 'better life' when we were growing up. I was bordering on a panic attack as I spoke, but I managed to remain controlled. I took deep breaths so my chokes didn't turn into panicked breaths and I started again whenever I needed to. He stood and listened for what seemed like forever. I told him everything – well, everything that I could, because I know now that I have blocked many things out along the way due to the horrific feelings I had.

I felt that he believed me. He stood up and as he was

leaving said, 'I am going to see your brothers and sister – if they tell me what you have, I will leave her, but I'll also not see you again, because if I allowed these things to happen, I don't deserve to be your dad.'

As I watched him leave, I knew then that I had lost him either way.

He did go to see my brothers and my sister, and they tell me they repeated my stories, along with their own, but he went home, and he married her. The sad truth is, I haven't ever seen or heard from him since that day nine years ago when he scaled my back gate. I cannot comprehend as a parent how you can just write your children off. I still go through stages where I question why my parents had four children. At times I feel so angry that they had both been selfish enough to produce us yet neither of them was ever committed enough to raise us for our whole lives – or to love and protect us. I try to let all the hurt, anger and hatred for him, my mum and Pam go or it would eat me up. I have spent too much money on therapy sessions where I cried over a broken childhood. Therapy sessions where I spent an hour just sobbing into a tissue while my amazing therapist explained and broke down what I was going through, how the people in charge of raising me as a child had failed me so badly.

Now, when anyone says to me, 'When your parents die it will all be too late' or, 'What I'd give to have my mum and dad alive again,' I think about how it is already too late. You don't stop being a parent when your child becomes an adult. I have needed my parents more in adulthood than I ever did when I was a child. I am still their child, and there should be something inside of them that makes them want to die for me, kill for me and love and protect me until the day they die – but it just isn't there. That switch that sits inside you when you become a parent never turned on for either of them, so I am done. I am a fatherless daughter, but I am absolutely at peace with that and, if anything, it makes me want what's right even more for my own children.

7

BABIES AND BINBAGS

However, there were more things I needed to do in my life to try and reach some kind of peace, and another major problem was my relationship with Tony. So, in May 2005, we split up. It was a Friday morning and we'd had a huge row because I'd asked for permission to go to the 'Run to the Sun' festival in Cornwall with some friends. He told me I wasn't going, but I hadn't left the house other than to go to work since Betsy had been born nine months earlier, and I just wanted one night to be me with my old girlfriends, to get drunk, laugh, and have no responsibility. The argument started as I was putting Betsy's clean washing away in her wardrobe and she sat on the rug not far from me.

'I'm going,' I told Tony.

'Watch what happens if you tell me you're going again.'

I knew. I knew exactly what would happen but that feeling I had of being controlled was so unjust, it was so unfair, that at the age of 23 I was having to ask my partner, have my first night out in almost a year and it was being refused, so I repeated the words to him.

'I'm going.'

The violence that rained down on me that day was horrific, all while my baby continued to sit nearby, sucking on her teething toys and babbling away to herself.

As soon as he left for work that night, I got Betsy and my things together then my brother John picked us up. I called the women's refuge in Exeter and they told me that they had a room for us. John dropped me at Exeter train station where I was met by a lady in a car who drove us to the safe house nearby. I was pumped full of adrenaline, fear and genuine sadness at what was happening.

I arrived at the refuge and felt so unwell. I kept being sick and couldn't eat. I blamed it on my anxiety and depression, but one of the ladies with me just kept looking at me as if she was thinking something through.

'How exactly do you feel?' she kept asking, but it was hard to answer as the vomiting wouldn't stop.

Finally, she left me with my head in the sink, but came back about fifteen minutes later. She'd gone out to buy me a pregnancy test.

She was right.

I was pregnant again.

When I saw the two blue lines appear, I genuinely thought my only option would be to kill myself. I was in such a bad place. A few days later, I went to the GP who referred me to the hospital and they confirmed that I was six weeks' pregnant. I felt absolutely devastated. I would spend ages in the refuge just watching Betsy, knowing I was carrying her sibling but facing the realisation that I just wasn't coping. I now weighed under six and a half stone and looked skeletal. I couldn't sleep and I couldn't see how I would manage with another baby. I spoke to my friends and family who all told me I would be mad to keep going with this pregnancy. In their eyes, my relationship with Tony was over and they were desperate to keep me away from him, so I booked a termination for the following Saturday.

On the day of the termination I went to Torbay Hospital with my sister. We sat in the waiting room and I was shaking with the emotion of it all. I did feel guilty but I also knew that there was no way I could justify bringing another baby into this mess. I still couldn't forget that Betsy was used to it now, as were her three older sisters. The four girls now didn't flinch when they heard screams and shouts and they continued to play alongside the violence they witnessed.

All of a sudden, Tony burst into the hospital screaming. He was shouting that I was a baby murderer and that I deserved to die. The whole waiting room just looked at me and him in total disbelief. No-one tried to stop him and he continued to rant and rave. Eventually security arrived and he was removed, but by now I was a mess – I was crying so hard that I wasn't actually crying, if that makes sense. It was like one of those cries children make when they really hurt themselves. The cry where there is no noise, just tears.

This continued until the anaesthetist told me he was unhappy to continue. I had to make this happen though. I knew in my head I had to go through with the termination, so I begged them to carry on, saying I was just upset with myself for getting into this situation. Eventually they agreed, but after the operation I was broken. I had never felt guilt like it. Last year I told Betsy the truth. I felt I had no option but to do this because her relationship with her dad had become so volatile. So I sat her down and explained to her my reasons and situation. She took my face in her hands, kissed my forehead and said 'I love you, Mum, don't ever think you have to explain yourself to me'.

After a few weeks of anger after the termination, Tony started begging me to go back to him – he said he was sorry, that he had changed, things would be different. He promised to leave the pub trade and get a normal job which meant we could be a family. I desperately missed my stepdaughters and I was carrying hideous guilt over the termination so. . . I went back. We had agreed to try one more time, moving house yet again, to give us another fresh start. I left the refuge pretending I wasn't going home but it was obvious to everyone what was happening. I guess they'd seen it all before. The women I met in there were amazing, we all swapped numbers and promised to stay in touch. One of them was from Birmingham, it was her seventeenth time in refuge and she had three babies to her partner. She was black and blue all over. She had been stabbed in the past, beaten with weapons, and repeatedly raped. I remember her eldest sons spitting at her and attacking her when they had tantrums – it was just devastating to watch. They had learned from the behaviour around them. Six months after I left the refuge, I saw her in Primark in Torquay with her children and partner. We both looked away like we didn't know each other, to keep her safe. That image has always stayed with me and I often wonder if she ever got away for good or if she's still there – or if she became a suicide statistic.

I met an elderly lady in the refuge too: a woman in her sixties who was wheelchair-bound due to ill-health. Her husband beat her every few months so she came to refuge for 'respite', as she called it, until he calmed down. She didn't even see that he was in the wrong; she just thought they needed a bit of time apart every so often. She was unable to conceive children when they were younger and, due to her illness, she needed him to care of her so she took the entire blame for his violence. It was heartbreaking. We never stayed in touch; there's something sad about that – after you spend so much time sharing stories and helping raise each other's children, you leave the refuge and never knew who returned to their partners, who became free, or whether any of them became another number on a coroner's report.

Upon returning home, things seemed better for a while, but I know now that this is part of the cycle. This was what is called the 'honeymoon period'. We moved away from the pub and Tony was now home in the evenings and around more at weekends. Soon, though, we began to argue. Sometimes I didn't fight back and I would try my hardest to be a good wife and mum, but it was draining. Other times I would cause the fights, I admit that. I was so trapped and unhappy that I would pick a fight knowing it would end with violence, just because I wanted unhappiness for us both rather than me alone. It was horrific. Volatile and abusive and poisonous, but it was normal, normal for me, normal for us; a continuing cycle that just went round and round for the next three years.

A year later and after more temporary splits, I became pregnant again.

I can't remember whether I was happy or sad or if the pregnancy was a mistake. I don't know why I don't remember such huge things, yet I remember silly small things like listening to Pink's album on repeat when I was driving to work or the little sport button that made my car go faster on my 2004-reg, baby blue Fiat Punto. I wanted to find out the gender of the baby, which we hadn't done with Betsy. Tony said 'No', but I begged and begged until he agreed. We went to the hospital with his mum and, upon having the scan, the sonographer told us we were having another little girl.

Tony flew into a rage. He started swearing and then stormed out of the scanning room. The sonographer asked if I was OK.

'If you hadn't found out the sex, he would have been fine,' Tony's mum said said. 'When the baby was born a girl, he would have loved her as soon as he had laid eyes on her, but you can't love a scan picture – what is he supposed to do? He'll have to go another four months knowing he isn't getting the boy he's desperate for.'

All my fault again.

I think the sonographer was in shock. It seems surreal looking back on that whole scenario now, but I can picture it all. Me thinking I had done something wrong and rather than being happy that I had a healthy baby girl inside me, I chased Tony through the hospital wards begging for forgiveness for conceiving a girl and promising him it would all be OK.

•

This labour started with the same swelling I'd had with Betsy. I was admitted to hospital and was induced. I kid you not, the contractions started within half an hour. I was on the level below the labour ward with my mum, sister and Tony. The midwives kept telling me I wasn't having contractions; that what I was feeling was pain from the inducing pill. I could tell they thought I was being dramatic and they refused me any pain relief, so I made Tony go to Boots and buy a TENS machine. The pain quickly became unbearable and my sister went to get the nurses. As I was in a ward that wasn't for labouring women, there were families visiting new mums and other pregnant women with issues, but no-one was in labour. Except me. It was busy, and by now I was writhing around the bed, throwing back the sheets while screaming, 'It's coming!' My mum went into full-blown panic as she saw the head, and, all of a sudden, loads of midwives appeared and ran with my bed up to the labour ward . . . only I didn't make it that far.

The baby arrived in the lift after about eighteen minutes, after a few goes on the gas and air.

Tony returned from Boots clutching a TENS machine, just in time to meet his fifth daughter.

Mum chose her name, Tallulah-Belle. She was 7 lb 10 oz and another perfect bundle of joy that I loved as much as her sister. I had no complications and went home the following day.

I don't remember suffering PND with Tallulah, but then, I don't remember much from any of that time, which makes me feel really shit. I went back to work six weeks later and Tony's mum raised all five girls while Tony and I were pretty much absent. Tony's mum was an amazing grandma and still is, but in my view she is his biggest victim. When he would lose his temper and I would call her for help, she would say things like, 'Don't answer him back, you will make him worse,' or, 'Just make him a cup of tea and say you're sorry and he will calm down.' I don't believe anyone should be actively encouraged to put up with it. I hated her for it.

To get through my relationship, I blamed the way Tony's mum had raised him for his behaviour. Of course, I see now that this is wrong: his actions are his alone and she just acted how she thought best; it was all she knew from her own relationships. As their grandma, I believe she has the girls' best interests at heart.

Life was no different for a while really – until it was.

On 27th December 2010, I left for the Next sale at 5 am. I queued in the cold for what seemed like hours. It was absolutely heaving and, while I was fighting other shoppers in the crowds, I heard a text ping and my phone vibrate. I ignored it and carried on shopping. When I walked back through the front door just before 8 am that morning, Tony was on the sofa with my three stepdaughters and Betsy, while Tallulah was still upstairs in her cot, asleep.

'Did you get my text?' he snapped.

'No,' I replied.

He immediately lost his temper.

Apparently, he had a headache and he had texted to ask me to go and buy him some paracetamol. I hadn't read the text so I hadn't bought him paracetamol, and this was all it took.

Right there and then, something clicked inside me. I don't know if it was watching Betsy quickly run upstairs so she wouldn't see what she knew was about to happen, or if it was my middle stepdaughter, who was now ten years old, repeatedly jumping and punching her dad in the back while screaming how much she hated him for what he was doing to me. I don't know if it was my baby stepdaughter, now nine years old, crouched behind the sofa knowing what was coming. I don't know if I knew I had one sleeping baby upstairs who I was determined to make a change for. I don't know if it was all this put together but something happened that day where I knew. It was different to all the other times I had left – this time I knew it was for good.

It went the same way it always did. I said I was leaving and told the girls to get their shoes on. He said I wasn't going anywhere; he locked the front door and hid the keys while things began spiralling more and more. He told the girls to ignore me being silly and everything would calm down. I told him calmly to let us go or I would smash my way out of the house. He knew right then that I was done and he knew that he had gone way too far.

He arranged for his ex-partner to collect the three elder girls while I took Betsy and Tallulah to my mum's. This was something she was ordered to do regularly when an incident occurred and Tony wanted them taken away from the house. I arrived at my mum's at 8.30 am. She saw the state of me and just cried. We had done this so many times, me arriving with the kids in tow, her crying, begging me to leave and telling me she feared I would end up dead. I'd always remain silent unless I was re-assuring the kids. She was so used to it, but this time I was adamant it was over. Usually Tony would arrive and when Mum didn't let him in, he would scream threats at her through her letterbox and windows and I would feel such guilt and panic that I would just apologise to Mum and go home to face the music. This time, though, Mum called John immediately – this was something we hadn't had to do since I had gone into refuge years earlier – and he arrived minutes later. I could see in his eyes that he was devastated, but I could also see he was tired of this routine. As calm as ever, he placed a wad of notes on Mum's coffee table.

'There's three grand there,' he said. 'You can have it on the condition you use it for a home for you and the girls and you never, ever go back.'

It was a lifeline.

My sister came and collected Betsy and Tallulah while I got cleaned up and made the decision to call the police. They arrived shortly after and began speaking to me. They do this interview where they have to ask you twenty-eight questions in relation to domestic abuse. One of the officers was a guy from my old school and I was mortified. I had left that school and town under a black cloud and now, coming face to face with him years later, I looked like I was in a worse state than back then. He was so sweet to me, and made such an effort to help me 'see the light', but I remember wanting to scream at him that I wasn't a scumbag. I had a good job, a company car, I was a decent person, a good mum, but, instead I just sat there in shame, utterly mortified at what he must have thought.

I remember feeling so ashamed when I was asked the questions, which are really intrusive and embarrassing. Now that I help women in my situation, I understand the purpose those questions serve and how important they are to build a case, but back then, I was just so disappointed in myself. It made everything much more real. My mum was sobbing while listening to me and I just wanted to curl up and die. It was the same self-hate I'd felt when I let Martin down.

The police agreed that, due to the situation they would return to my home and be present while I collected my belongings.

I took my clothes, the girls' clothes, and a single mattress. I left behind everything else I had spent years working my ass off for. The whole time I was packing my things, he sat on the sofa trying to tell anyone who would listen how sorry he was – I guess, in his head, he was, he always was, but 'sorry' when you are in a relationship like that means nothing after a while.

I was back to having my life in binbags – six this time – and as I headed away, I knew that I was about to hit rock bottom in order to climb back up again.

●

I now see this phase of my life as a turning point. It had just gotten so bad. I was worn down. It's the point at which I could take no more – and I started to feel that I deserved to be saved.

● Looking back on this, I would probably advise people to always follow their heart. If I'd followed mine, I never would have gone back for seconds with my dad and our relationship. He broke my heart before any other man got the chance to, years before I should have experienced heartbreak from any man, and because I listened to someone else, I went back and endured it all again. Sometimes we walk into fire because we want what other people have, even though we know we're not going to get it, when actually it's better to just keep walking the opposite way.

● Learn from others every day – it's something I struggled to do. Look at the woman who's been beaten in the refuge and do anything and everything you can to stop yourself from turning into her. If you are her, learn from that too; learn from the women who have moved on from that refuge and stayed away. The ones who did get their lives and their freedom back and convince yourself you can be them.

● Things WILL work out. No matter how bad they seem, how much of a shit situation you have got yourself into, and how many toxic people you're surrounded by, you have to keep hope and you have to keep going through it all, because if you have an idea of how you want your life to look, if you have that dream, you just need to plan, in baby steps day by day.

8

STARTING OVER

I moved into a flat which was an absolute shithole. There was no central heating, and it had previously belonged to an old lady who had suffered from incontinence before her family had taken her to a care home to be looked after. The smell was horrendous and the décor was appalling: the bathroom was carpeted with cream shag-pile, which I imagine had been laid about thirty years earlier – it was spectacular really, I can't even begin to describe the colour or stench of it. I had nothing, apart from a single mattress, a blow-up bed and two double quilts my mum had given me.

That night I saw New Year's Eve in with my daughters and my two youngest stepdaughters. We played Scrabble and ate Domino's pizza, we had a bedsheet up at the window and we all slept together on the mattresses on the lounge floor. I remember watching all four of them snooze around me. I didn't have a pot to piss in, I had spent the past 24 hours clearing used needles off the tops of my kitchen cupboards which had been left there by the previous tenants (who, my neighbours told me, had been evicted due to their heroin addiction), and I had no idea how I was going to make anything right for them ever again, but I knew that somehow, this surely had to be the beginning of my happiness.

The next few months were horrific. It may well have been coincidental but it was at that time that my mum was investigated for benefit fraud by the council, and my company car got keyed, twice. Tony rang my sister several times with unfounded allegations about her husband. Again, the guilt sat heavy in me as people continued to suffer, I believed, because of my life choices and, while my family all continued to support me, I knew that they had endured ten years of this man in my life – which ultimately kept me stronger to prove to them I wouldn't go back.

As much as I knew I had made the right choice, I felt broken. As I explained earlier, my therapist says that because of abandonment issues in my childhood, I struggle to cope with being alone, and I am OK with admitting that now because I know it's not my fault. I hope when I do struggle, it makes other women see that we are not weak because of it. I see some of my closest friends rock the shit out of being single mommas and they're absolutely fine with being by themselves, whereas I hated it. I felt so alone.

I hated not having a family unit. I hated not having someone to look after me even though the reality was I had never really been looked after. I panicked every night and day that I would never meet anyone to love me or my babies.

Every other weekend, the girls went to their dad. I would sit in the flat and cry – big, fat sobs which would lead into a panic attack. I would also cry when the girls were asleep at sleep at night and I was awake, alone. That was the word that seemed to just flow through everything – *alone*. My friends rallied round as much as they could and while they were with me, I felt much better, but they had their own lives and families and it just wasn't practical for them to be there all the time.

Over the following year I went on a few shitty dates. I quite liked one guy, we saw each other for a couple of months and I invited him along to a big BBQ I went to with some friends at a local pub, but the following week it was my birthday and he bought me a Supernanny book, clearly letting me know that he thought my kids were arseholes, so that relationship ended up being short-lived.

I then met up with someone called Sam who I had gone out with at school; we were a couple for about six months before I left Brixham when I was fifteen. Sam had also come out of a really difficult situation and was a bit lost, and I think he was as desperate as I was to settle down. Immediately, he wanted to take me and the girls on. He was a good, decent man.

Sam worked away from Monday to Friday, but, when he was home, he spoiled us with love and gifts and he was definitely good for us. But then a few months in I had a moment of clarity where I knew it wasn't right, and when Sam came home on the Friday I explained how I felt. He said he would give me space, and left me alone . . . and I missed him, just not in a way where you're in love but in a way you miss a companion, a friend. He was my friend and I loved him, so after a day apart I again convinced myself I would make things work. By now, I also knew that I absolutely hated being alone and stupidly I allowed it all to move way too quickly with him. Rather than having therapy, learning to love myself again and seeing that I could actually cope on my own, I decided that a full-on hardcore relationship right now was just what I needed – so in I jumped.

Pretty soon, I was pregnant. I convinced myself I was happy, really happy – and I couldn't wait to have a pregnancy where I would be looked after and safe. After a scan I was informed there was no heartbeat. I had to wait seven days, then be scanned again in case the sonographer was incorrect and the baby was, in fact, healthy. Seven days later I went back but there was still no heartbeat. The happiness was over, just like that. It was so sudden, so devastating. My baby was surgically removed under general anaesthetic the following week.

I continued to try for another baby, blaming my unhappiness on the miscarriage and, a few months later, I fell pregnant again. Things were going well and then it was like déjà vu – another scan, no heartbeat, and another operation.

I know that at this point I wasn't easy to live with. I was hormonal, desperate for a baby, and I believed that, as soon as I had one, it would be the answer to everything. Looking back I can see how ridiculous that was, but I'd lost two babies in such quick succession when I'd thought things were finally getting better, so it seems almost predictable that I would start to make connections that weren't there.

I became pregnant again a few months later but spent the whole nine months in a state of panic as I thought I would lose the baby. I dreaded the visits to the midwife, where she would listen for a heartbeat – I didn't sleep for days leading up to the scans. Thankfully, everything seemed to be going well until, six weeks before I was due, the midwife told me that the baby was breech. I began going in weekly to see if the baby had moved, but it hadn't. They then asked if I wanted an appointment where the doctor would 'turn' the baby so I could avoid a caesarean section and try to have another vaginal birth. I agreed to this but went home and began researching on

YouTube what actually happens. I worked out that the doctor actually manipulates the baby around your belly using lots of movements, almost forcing the baby into a non-breech position. It looked really uncomfortable and I worried whether it would stress the baby.

I arrived the following week for the appointment, and, upon having a scan, I was told the umbilical cord was wrapped around the baby's neck and there was minimal fluid surrounding it. The doctor said he was happy to try and still move the baby; however, the risks were now higher and there was every chance it could flip back around immediately after being turned. I was beyond nervous but I was also worried about having a caesarean section. It would mean Tallulah would be starting her induction days at primary school just after the birth and I wouldn't be able to drive her there and back, so the shit-mum guilt hit me – starting school was a huge thing in her little life and she would feel so left out. I couldn't do it, though; I couldn't go through with the attempts to shift the baby. As soon as he did one movement to give me an indication of what he would be doing, I almost hurled all over him with the pressure I felt, so I packed up my stuff and went home to wait for my invite letter for my first caesarean section.

I arrived at the hospital on 23rd August 2013 at 8 am to be informed I was last on the list. I waited for a while and a nurse came in to insert my cannula, before I was finally taken into theatre just before midday. I have never gone into theatre awake before and I felt like I had died. Everything is so white that your eyes hurt and it just reminded me of how it would be going to heaven, and I don't even know if I believe in heaven. I would describe a caesarean section as someone washing up in your belly, there was a lot of pulling and pushing and I could see my shoulders juddering about from being moved but there was no pain at all.

It seemed like very shortly after it began, I was handed my 6 lb 13 oz baby girl whom I named Edie, chosen again by my mum. Immediately, I needed to be sick. It was the same sick as a drunk sick on the way home in the back of a taxi where you feel like the alcohol is poisoning your body and you need to get it out. I started retching but I was lying flat on my back and couldn't get it all out. I was totally numb, so unable to get myself up and I started really panicking. I was trying to stick my fingers down my throat but I had the machines attached to me and the nurses were holding my hands down. In the end I vomited over myself and I began crying because I was panicking so much.

My friend Hannah was quite a pro at having caesarean sections and she told me I would be allowed home the day after giving birth as long as I passed enough fluid, so I drank and drank and drank. I went to the extremes of drinking as if I had been in the Sahara for three days without any liquid. The following day the nurses followed me to the toilet to take a wee in the cardboard piss pot and I couldn't stop. I had lost all ability to stop pissing and it just kept coming and coming! It even went over the side of the bowl. I was trying to shuffle back towards the toilet but the pain was horrific so I just continued to wee, all over the toilet floor. It was like a river and I was absolutely mortified. It worked, though, because straight afterwards they got me changed, packed my bag full of painkillers and sent me home.

The pain of the caesarean section was like nothing I had known before and getting up with the baby in the night is such hard work because when you wake to their cries, you forget what you've just endured and you go to sit up but it just knocks you back – you forget that when you pull your body up to sit, you use all the tummy muscles that have been cut open. When you cough, sneeze, or move slightly, it wrecks. You have a day where the pain seems less so you do more, maybe take baby for a quick stroll or run the vacuum round, but you then pay for it the next day when you can't move at all. I remember the surgeon explaining to me that because it was such a common procedure, people forget that it is actually a really big operation. She tried to show me how your tummy muscles knit together really intricately, then they are sliced through! For it to repair takes time, and for that to happen, you have to rest, but that's easier said than done when you are a mum with a newborn, and other kids to add to the equation. I remember finding the recovery so much harder than I had with my first two babies. If I was to have another and I got the choice, I would choose popping them out my fandango any day.

I was postnatally depressed again, but, at the time, I was adamant I wasn't. By now I had a huge, beautiful home, lots of friends visiting me, was financially stable, my boyfriend wasn't a bastard – so I couldn't work out why I cried in secret every day. I would sob in the shower, knowing that no-one would hear me, and all of those feelings of being desperate, lonely and unhappy came flooding back.

In the end, I cried in front of Sam, often. And he was helpless, he was helpless because he didn't understand either and I suppose that just created a bigger distance between us.

Sam was, by now, working away all the time. His bosses had no interest in family life and would expect him to stay away over weekends as well by now, going as far as the Isle of Wight or Holland at a moment's notice. When he returned, I would cause arguments because I suppose I felt he was still carefree and didn't understand how hard things were for me running this tiny female army while he could come and go as he pleased. Actually, I imagine all he wanted was to be at home with us.

By the time Edie was four months old I decided

I couldn't be with Sam anymore. I knew, through the deepest bouts of depression, that this wasn't meant to be. I knew he deserved someone who loved him more than I did, who wanted all the things I couldn't make myself feel. When Sam came home I told him I loved him, but I wasn't *in* love with him. I offered for him to live with us as I didn't have the right to take the three girls from him and he was a brilliant dad/stepdad, but I didn't want our relationship. I just felt I couldn't do it. He did not want to stay under those conditions, so he packed his things and went to his friends in Blackpool before moving out completely a few days later.

For me right now, today, after living through the pain of having my heart broken and breaking someone else's heart, if I had the choice, I would choose to have my heart broken all day long. I don't think you ever get over the guilt and devastation that comes with ripping someone's heart out because of your own choices. It sits with you always, years down the line, even after they heal and move on. When you have your heart broken, you do eventually get over it and despite at the time it being the worst lesson to learn, it's just that, a lesson learned.

Things became pretty horrific after I made the choice to end that relationship. I lived in a small town where I was now widely hated by a whole raft of people for upsetting one of the most popular, well-liked blokes in it.

Facebook has a lot to answer for in my life – it led me

back to Joshua around this time (remember him? Hannah's older gorgeous brother?). I was at my very worst and we had been speaking on Facebook for a few months. He had the same sense of humour, which is what I love about his sister. He made me feel like me again, before I had the girls, before I started making shitty life-changing mistakes. Josh had two sons whom he idolised, and he was a police officer in our town.

I started falling for him hard – and I panicked. I can only describe it as the same feelings I had when I used to dream about marrying Mark Owen when I looked at my Take That posters plastered all over my room when I was about twelve years old! That kind of teenage girl crush where you dream about marrying someone you will never meet. I started thinking about Josh as soon as I woke up; I was checking his profile a million times a day, and, in general, just freaking myself out being a weird stalker. I was also breastfeeding a tiny baby, and I had two other daughters I needed to focus on. I needed to sort myself out about going back to work so I could pay the bills on the huge house I could no longer afford the rent on, pay the finance on the car I could no longer afford to drive, and pay everything else that I now had full responsibility for. But, if I am totally honest, I didn't think for one minute Josh would be interested in someone like me and I knew I was messing my own head up more than anything.

I decided I was being a total weirdo, so, to sort my life out, I decided to block Josh on Facebook. A few hours later, he messaged me on Instagram asking why I had blocked him. I felt sick that he had even noticed, let alone think of what to answer. I decided to stick with what my big brother had always told me, that 'honesty was the best policy' and roll with the truth. I wrote back the most rambling, ridiculous shit-filled message about how my body thought it was in love with him but it wasn't, I just had crazy hormones buzzing about from having a baby. I told him I was overtired and perhaps had a touch of PND, therefore I was going to book myself a doctor's appointment so he could make my brain better, perhaps with some medication; then, once it was and I stopped feeling like I was in love with him, I would unblock him on social media and just be normal again!

He replied immediately.

'Meet me now,' it said.

I had only ever left Edie once for a few hours by this point and I knew my mum would wonder what was going on if I said I was going out. I told her I was nipping to the doctors for five minutes to grab a prescription and, as Edie had only just gone down, I would leave her to sleep.

I went out the door stinking of stale milk. I hadn't washed my hair for three days and I probably could have knitted my armpit hair. I had no idea what I was thinking as I got in my car and started driving towards him, but I knew I was an absolute mess. I certainly expected Josh to be really confident when I saw him whereas, I, on the other hand, was by now a nervous wreck.

I met him at the top of a crossroads close by and, as I pulled up, I remember wondering if we were going for a walk, or if I should get in his car, or if he was going to get into mine – then I looked round my car and it resembled a mobile skip. I was mortified, so quickly jumped out and got into his. He was visibly shaking. His hands were all jittery and he had a bottle of water he kept sipping from nervously.

I can picture every detail that day.

His car had one of those tree air fresheners hanging on the mirror called 'Black Ice'. That smell today would bring back all of those feelings, I imagine; it's funny how smells have the power to do that. I remember his car was immaculate. I remember thinking that I was pleased I'd made the choice to go to his because if he'd seen the state of mine, he would have got straight back out and driven off!

He looked so nervous, frightened almost. He kept flipping the lid on his bottle of water and it was beyond awkward.

We both giggled nervously.

'Do you want to go for a walk?' he asked.

I said 'yes' and got out the car. Within seconds, it started to hail. Josh grabbed my hand and we ran to a sort of wooden bunker, wet through. We stood under the bunker to shelter from the rain and I could see that his hands were still really shaking.

Then, he turned around and held my face with both of his hands and kissed me.

I'd like to say how romantic it was but it really wasn't! I looked like utter shit and he was a shaking, silent mess. I had no idea whether he was going in for a peck or a snog, and I thought I was going to hurl with the nerves I had, so it was all a bit of a fuck up to be honest. I didn't understand what was going on, so I started rambling on that I was crazy. I kept telling him I had three kids by two men and repeatedly pointed out everything that would put him off because I was in shock that he was saying all this stuff to me and it was clear he wasn't aware of what a liability I was . . . and, and, and . . .

He kissed me again.

'I'm in love with you,' he said. 'I'll wait for you. I understand that things are tough and that Edie is tiny and that everything is really shit and raw – but I'll wait for you because I love you.'

He was adamant that he didn't want to pressure me into anything more than what we had, but that he would wait, years if he had to. He didn't want to have sex, he didn't want to see me in person if it made things difficult.

He was happy just to keep chatting and messaging for as long as I needed.

Fuck, I thought, *what's happening now?*

●

I suppose, reflecting upon this part of my life, I almost feel grateful that things got so bad, because it showed me when they were getting better – and they did. Each week I made improvements, no matter how small, and felt happier.

● Being a single parent is the hardest job in the world. When you're doing it while not in a good place, I would advise you to keep busy, especially on a Sunday. For some reason, it felt like my loneliest day, so try to be with your family and friends. It's better to be silent or sobbing with someone holding your hand.

● It's crazy how your body changes with each new delivery to get the baby out of your body. My first birth was the most hideous labour, where I became extremely poorly afterwards, and my second one was so short she was born in the lift with very little pain relief and I was home the following day with no complications. But the caesarean section with Edie was a different experience again. No pregnancy or birth is the same, so if you have had horrendous experiences, don't let it put you off trying again because all of mine were so different!

● Break-ups are the most horrific things to endure when you have children. The heartache, devastation and guilt that take over are unbelievable and there are periods where you think it will never end or get easier . . . but it does. It's all just time, and it passes much more quickly than you might imagine when you're in the middle of the shit.

9

US AGAINST THE WORLD

Over the next few months, life was beyond vile. It didn't seem to have calmed down at all. Sam had moved on to new relationships with other people while I met Josh for coffee out of town occasionally, but he was also going through a tough time with his ex-wife and trying to prioritise his sons, so we just messaged and spoke lots without seeing each other much.

A few months later, it was my birthday. Sam was having Edie overnight for the first time since we had separated, and Josh took me away to Cheltenham for the night. We talked a lot on the way up there and I decided I didn't want to keep us a secret anymore. I had never had any time away from Edie and only a few nights a month without Betsy and Lula when they were with their paternal family. So, given that Josh's job was really demanding, seeing each other alone was proving to be difficult. While away, we agreed to start doing things together with our kids 'as friends' and they started getting to know each other. Unfortunately, the town we lived in was extremely small, and within a few hours of us being in Cheltenham, I had received hate messages about being away with Josh.

We returned the following day and, from then on, we were about to experience hell like I had never known. Within ten days of people finding out about our relationship, Josh was arrested by his own colleagues under horrendous allegations. Although these proved to be false, he spent eight hours sat in a police cell and, over the month, he was subjected to both internal and external investigations and removed from public-facing duties. At that time, Josh was due to be awarded a bravery medal for rescuing a woman from a house during an extremely dangerous domestic violence situation – her perpetrator was given a lengthy custodial sentence for this incident – but he was informed that the award would be put on hold pending the outcome of the investigations.

I received calls from Children's Services, who had received allegations that I was abusing my children, and my employer received calls saying I was stealing money from them. I can't prove if anyone was behind these events, or who that could be, but Josh and I were now being attacked in the most cowardly ways by a whole town of people, me to my face and him all over social media. Public statuses were written about us, and pictures of us and my children were put up. People we had never met would comment that I should have my womb removed so I couldn't have any more children. Someone said that Josh should be paid a visit in a dark alley and we were told that we should both have our children taken away. It was truly the dark side of social media. More surprisingly, people we did know and people who were supposed to be our friends were also responding to these comments, liking them and sharing them, which meant that this toxic venom spread far and wide. It was us against a whole town, it seemed.

Edie's father and I ended up in Family Court twice during the first two years of Edie's little life. During that time, my ex-partner and father of my youngest daughter, Sam, and Josh's ex-wife and mother to his sons, decided to embark on a relationship. Sam became the stepfather to Josh's sons and he moved in with them. You couldn't make it up.

All of the children were bewildered and confused. My older girls couldn't understand why their once amazing stepdad, who had loved them so much, was now living with my new partner's ex-partner. It was beyond belief and left us in shock.

Josh and I were about to embark on two years of utter hell.

Before Sam and I were due in court, I agreed to give him some supervised access to Edie. He had, by now, ended his relationship with Josh's ex and seemed to be trying to make an effort to be in Edie's life. I'd had a really long telephone conversation with Sam from my work phone where he was so upset, and I broke for the situation he was now in. With Christmas around the corner I wanted him to spend some time with Edie in the hope that things would become better for us all. One of my closest friends, Karen, agreed to supervise the access on Christmas Eve for five hours at her house. Edie loved Karen and was used to spending time with her children as they would sleep at our house most weekends, and Betsy would sleep at theirs a lot of the time too. We saw each other most days. When Karen dropped Edie home, she said it had gone well and she kept going on about what an amazing dad he was. I found that quite strange given that she'd seen me go through hell. Still, it was positive, Edie was happy, and it was progress.

The following day, Christmas Day, was also Karen's birthday. I called her first thing to wish her a 'Happy Birthday' and to see if she was OK. I had taken her kids out the day before to buy presents for her from them. She answered the phone and, almost immediately, told me she had spent the night with Sam. I remember I didn't say much, I think I was in shock.

When I put the phone down, I told Josh and he was really angry – Karen and Josh had grown up together, and he loved her mum and dad to bits. Josh doesn't argue with people. He isn't nasty and he doesn't entertain any kind of conflict – he says it how it is, calmly and rationally and that's that. He doesn't scream and shout, he just makes his point and he's always fair. What he was hurt about is that, because of what we had endured together, we had cut ourselves off from most people. We had almost become recluses and we didn't have many friends at that point because the drama that surrounded us was so humiliating that we were embarrassed. We'd also stopped trusting people because we had been let down time and time again. The only person we really spoke to about the whole situation was Karen – Josh as well as me – and she was understanding of that. She didn't judge us, she supported us, and I think Josh was genuinely hurt because he considered Karen to be one of our very best friends and all five of our children loved her.

At that time Karen had a mouth infection and she hated dentists so I had arranged to take her for her appointment a few days later. She stopped calling me after the bombshell about spending the night with Sam, so I decided to drive to her house and sort things out with her. When I pulled up, Sam's car was on the drive . . . and the next day and the day after that. It was clear that they were now living together.

By this time, I had run out of people to supervise contact between Sam and Edie, so I agreed to do it myself. We went to a soft play area every other Saturday for three hours. After a few weeks I was to leave him and Edie alone for a few hours – I was then in charge of allowing more access as and when it was appropriate. Edie loved Sam immediately and it was clear to me he idolised her. They look so alike and they have the same features: their hands, their feet, the same face when they're tired and they both sleep deeply with their mouths open. When I saw them together, it broke me that she had missed out on so much time with her daddy due to the shit that goes on between adults.

Over time Edie's contact with her dad became more regular and she now stays at his house every Wednesday plus every other Saturday, and if he wants extra time that's also fine. Sam is still with Karen and they're really happy. I'm not ever going to be the person that says, 'She was never my friend to do that to me' because I believe she was my friend. She was a really good friend, one who loved me, looked out for me, and wanted the best for me. She was like an aunt to mine and Josh's children and she supported me when things were bad, so when this happened I was heartbroken. I won't be the person that says I didn't care because, actually, I did care. Her choice hasn't made me love or question any of my other friends any less. I still love them all as much and as hard as I can. Karen was my friend, one of my very best, but I felt upset and disappointed by her choice of partner. She is an amazing stepmum to Edie, so it doesn't hurt me anymore. Sometimes, I find an old picture of us, or a card, or a memory, and it makes me question how it ever came to this, but, ultimately, we're all OK and happy. If a lost friendship had to happen to lead to this, then so be it.

Now that we all get on, Edie is the happiest, most secure little girl because she is loved by both sets of parents and stepparents. She doesn't hear negativity and she is allowed to love. She sees her daddy come into our house and chat, and she sees Karen and I getting on when I drop her to their house. Edie is allowed to tell me she has a second mummy, and she is allowed to call Josh her daddy too because that's what she wants. That's what makes her happy, so that's what we do. After years of turmoil, I am finally at peace with how things have turned out. I just wish we could all get on with our exs like this but life, and the page, has taught me that it just isn't the case very often.

While I was fighting Sam, Josh was also fighting his ex-partner over their two boys. His eldest son was eight years old at the time and would tell Josh all sorts of worrying things about the situation at home. He then stopped talking altogether. Both boys totally changed, we felt, and became really withdrawn.

No matter how many times Josh voiced his concerns to professionals, it seemed nothing could change. The school said it needed permission from the courts to allow them to step in and the courts did not respond to Josh's emails. So it continued, and continued. It was utterly draining and heartbreaking.

Josh didn't sleep a full night throughout these two years. I would wake to find him sobbing downstairs. He was convinced something bad would happen to the boys.

We naively borrowed tens of thousands of pounds to pay for solicitors and barristers to represent us, and, other than going to work, neither of us left the house without each other. There were nights, whole nights, when we just wouldn't sleep. We were so unwell with anxiety that we couldn't eat, we lost so much weight, and every day we faced a new public status or challenge online. It was so stressful.

It was relentless. I know that we're not the only ones it happens to and that making a patchwork family is one of the hardest things in the world, but there were times when I just couldn't see any light at the end of the tunnel and wondered how we would ever get through it. There were days where Josh and I couldn't bear to be apart from one another. There were days when we just couldn't bring ourselves to open the post in case it was more bad news or answer another call from a withheld number because we knew it would be something else that would devastate us, but the reality is you have to. You have to keep going, and hoping that it will get better.

A friend sent me this and I think it's beautiful, so now

seems like a good time to put it in, just to remind anyone out there going through this sort of shit, just what it is you are fighting for . . .

So, what is a patchwork family?

Families thrown together in the aftermath of a distressing or harmful break-up? Perhaps. Families brought together after years of compromising and understanding? That's us.

I find myself in a very unusual but extremely satisfying situation, where two families have been brought together as one.

My family consists of me, my wife Sarah, my son Jackson, who is nearly 13, and our son Alfie, who is 7.

When Alfie was two, his mum Sarah and I made the difficult decision to live our lives separately; she was young and had dreams of university and certainly wasn't ready for the reality of family life. It was hard, very hard. I missed my boy more than I ever thought possible, but I knew I had done the right thing. I was brought up in a home with arguments and sometimes violence and, although it would never have got to that, the tension between us when we were together was unbearable and there was no way that I was going to let my son be a part of that.

Life was tough. Every decision I made regarding Alfie was met with controversy – having to liaise with someone when you have so much resentment clouded every judgement I had to make. Before long, there was another man in Sarah's life. Another father figure spending the time with my son that I should have been. Resentment turned to anger; I found it so hard to control my emotions. Every time I used to drop him home, I would fight to hold back the tears, quite unsuccessfully most of the time.

Not long after, I met Sarah Number 2 – this woman was perfect. She adored me and adored Alfie. I had found someone who would do anything for either of us. We were a family.

As years passed, things got better. Initially, I was very unfair to Sarah's partner. He was caught up in a situation through no fault of his own and had been nothing but polite and courteous to me. In fact, over time, I had come to realise that this guy who I had resented so much at the start was actually the best father figure I could have ever wished for Alfie. Also, with the relationship between me and Sarah, he was often the voice of reason at times of adversity and conflict; he was the glue that pulled our once-damaged relationship back together for the sake of our son.

So often, people have been amazed at the relationship that has developed between our families. Much praise has been given to Sarah and me for the harmonious lives that we live, but we are not the ones who should be praised. Sarah's partner has been understanding and trusting, he has let me be the dad and never stood in my way. Without that, our lives would never have been how they are now. However, the person who deserves more praise than anyone is my new partner. She has been so understanding from day one. I mean, how many girlfriends would support you and understand whenever you wanted to go around your ex's house, or even stay over on Christmas Eve to be able to wake up and see your little boy's face in the morning? I don't think I'll ever understand how hard it must have been for her, but she stood by me and every decision I had to make for the good of my child.

And now we have a boy together! Another son! I couldn't be happier. A brother to Alfie, who, despite initially thinking my partner was going to give birth to a dinosaur, was over the moon with his new sibling.

Life has settled down nicely for us all. The birth of James was shortly followed by the marriage of Sarah and her partner, and soon after they had a little girl, Chloe. I feel this was the time that brought us all together. Chloe was diagnosed with a very rare type of cancer when she was only a few months old, and it devastated us all. I would have done anything to make it better for them but I felt helpless, they were going through so much pain. But, by some divine miracle, she pulled through and has turned into a beautiful, funny little girl who is like the daughter I've never had.

Chloe regularly stays with us and her brothers, as James does at their house. I sometimes find myself looking at my family, my partner on her phone, the boys bickering because Alfie has just thrown James into a fiery furnace on Minecraft, and Chloe snuggled up to me on the sofa talking absolute rubbish, and think how lucky I am to have such a beautiful family and how things have turned out.

Last year, we got married, my boys at my side, Chloe as our beautiful flower girl, and Sarah and her husband as our witnesses. Ridiculous, some might think, but I believe that it's amazing. Sarah is due to have another little boy any day now and we can't wait to welcome him into our family.

Every one of us has played a part. Compromises, understanding, sacrifices, trust and love.

What is a patchwork family? I'd like to think that if you looked it up there would be a picture of us – and I couldn't be happier.

●

The stress, the heartache and the complications of being a patchwork family can sometimes feel overwhelming – but you can make it work and you will get there. Here are a few tips I would give to anyone battling it out:

- Family Court is something I am asked about daily. It is a daunting process and while Women's Aid works tirelessly to change how the courts do things, there are still huge improvements that need to be made. Some judges save worlds, while others seem to make choices that devastate childhoods. What I will say is you CAN self-represent. It is daunting but I couldn't afford a solicitor so I did represent myself and I was OK. The court process is explained by CAFCASS and you will get through it. Please don't panic about it all. There is nowhere near enough awareness of it and because of that it frightens people.

- It's not forever. As difficult as it is to fight with an ex-partner and to feel beyond hurt at their actions and choices, it isn't forever. It feels like it is; it feels like you will always be drowning in misery and everyone you thought you could trust can't be trusted, but actually, it's not that bad. Time heals, and with healing you do forget, forgive and move on. I promise.

● If your new partner has children then watch what type of parent they are. Personally, I would rather be irritated by a guy who wanted to bring his kids along to everything we did than not see them. Children need good role models. They need parents whose love will help them thrive, and I believe that how a person treats their child from a previous relationship says a huge amount about them.

10

BECOMING A FAMILY

When something happens now that reminds us of that time and we talk about it, we sometimes laugh, sometimes I still cry; a lot of the time Josh will give my leg a squeeze and my forehead a kiss and I know it's his way of saying 'We made it' and really, both of us have no idea how we did. Day and night for two years, we fought a town full of people who held such venom and poison for us and it was relentless. It affected our families and at times I used to think it would end up being the death of Josh's mum.

What I also remember from that time is how many people let us and our children down. People who we thought would have been there for us weren't and that taught me a huge lesson: never take opinion or get involved in situations you don't know enough about, because the effects can be truly damaging.

Josh's workforce should have protected him and

looked after him, but they didn't. The police, the people you think are there to protect you, actually did everything *but* protect him, or that is how we saw it. All these people who could have helped make a shitty situation a bit better, just made it worse, and it made me question the world and how people behave and act. I was determined that one day I would help to change it.

We arrived at the final court hearing in July 2015 and Josh was awarded full custody of both boys and their mum was given supervised access in a contact centre. But things didn't get better as we had hoped.

Some days I hated her, some days I could have physically hurt her when I thought of what the boys had been through, but mostly, I just wanted her to get some help which we felt she needed. When I listened to her last voicemail, I could hear how desperate she was. It broke me that she had two beautiful boys and an ex-partner who just wanted her to be OK, but it seemed she just felt so bad. She did not have enough support, in my opinion, and it was a hideous, sad situation – one I couldn't see getting any better.

We went back to court and it was decided the boys would live with Josh until they were eighteen.

The process was slow but I genuinely think the respite allowed the boys' mum to see things for what they were. Right now Sebastian understands more than Isaac because unfortunately he witnessed more and was of an age to understand it. This week the realisation has hit that Isaac is perhaps coming to an age where we need to be honest but actually we don't know what's more damaging; so Josh has engaged with a registered charity and asked for help to understand how best to protect his eight -year-old son going forward until hopefully his mum can play her part in caring for him again.

●

I get asked the question about our ex-partners so often by email and in my live shows. It's something you guys are extra inquisitive about and I understand it because I am the same with people. Things are better now with Edie's dad and the boys' mum, but it took a long time getting there and I won't lie – there are days when something comes into my head that they did, or I come across a CAFCASS report or court order, and those feelings re-emerge, but only for a short while, because I look at where we are now, and how happy and settled our children are. I want that to remain so I take some deep breaths. I do remember the shit times, but I realise how lucky we are to no longer be there – to have overcome it all – because some people never find that peace.

Unfortunately, it's not the same with Betsy and Tal-lulah's dad, Tony, which is a shame considering we split up almost a decade ago. You can't get on with everyone; there are some people in life who are just too hard to work alongside – and for me, he is one of them. I have come to the realisation that will probably never change. Every time I've tried to get along with him, it has backfired and it drained me so much that a few years ago, Josh took on the role of dealing with him. Josh manages the most horrid, awkward people in his job, he doesn't react to anything, he doesn't get wound up and never goes back for anyone who is trying to aggravate him, but shortly after he began contact with Tony to arrange his visits with the girls, he just felt that even he couldn't manage him. He was always drained after dealing with Tony, so we decided to no longer speak to him. He is blocked on both our phones so we don't receive the messages. He calls to speak to Tallulah from a withheld number whenever he wants to, and it's hard because occasionally we get a glimmer of a good dad. There will be no issues for months and you start to think that things are improving, then something happens, something as trivial as sending Tallulah without a jumper or the right shoes and we go back to square one. At the time of writing this I have just been shown a public Facebook status that someone who isn't involved has written about me saying what an evil person and a bad mother I am . . . all of which seems pointless trying to fight. It takes a lot of effort to not respond. But it's the best way. Josh has a guy he goes birding with who once said to me, 'You can't educate pork' and that saying has stuck with me ever since because it's true, you really can't.

Betsy's relationship with her dad is drastically different to Tallulah's – she isn't frightened of him when he loses his temper. She also has something inside her which I see inside me – the need to protect the people she loves and it burns in her fiercely, despite her being so young.

Tony's downfall, it seems to me, is that he learned nothing. I am told that he continues to speak badly of me to Betsy and Tallulah whereas I would never do that about him because of what I experienced in my own childhood. I also will not allow Betsy to speak about him negatively to Tallulah, so if she starts I ask her to go to her room where I follow and let her have a private rant to myself or Josh, away from little ears that look up to their big sister and want to be just like her. Betsy knows what her dad says is wrong. She idolises me as her mother; she has taken on that protector role with me no matter how many times I tell her it isn't how it should be – so, over time he has just driven her further away. She is also now of an age where she has the independence and knowledge to walk out of his house and get on a bus and tell me when he has started shouting, meaning that in the past year she has totally stopped seeing him. There is still a part of me that always hopes he will miss her so much that he will change for good, but right now, he seems to be still very much the same person that he was when we were together; she is at an age where things are tough for her, but he doesn't seem to see that; he doesn't see that, right now, she doesn't know if she's coming or going – her body is changing, she is a grown-up in a child's body. She needs people around her who understand all of that in order to parent her properly and he doesn't seem to get it at all; and I imagine he won't when it comes to Tallulah.

Right now with Tallulah, I just monitor how she is. At the moment, she is easy, she's laid-back and well-behaved so the six nights a month she sees him, he manages – and while she is happy and it's going well, I would never step in. It isn't my job to stop him being a father when he is a positive influence – if he wanted more involvement I would encourage that. However, he knows that the minute he upsets Tallulah I will be there, and I will protect her because it's a role as a child no-one took on for me, so I am super-aware as a mum and stepmum that we have to do it for our own children. Right now, Tony and I have managed contact without the use of Family Court. He has access to Tallulah every other weekend and on the Sunday in between she stays with his mum and it works well. There are times she doesn't want to go but mainly because she feels she's missing out on something I am doing with the boys or Betsy as they are always at home, But overall she enjoys going so there has been no need to have a court order in place.

Family Court is a daunting place; you see and hear things in the waiting rooms that make you question the world around you, and nothing was ever explained properly. Looking back now, Josh could have self-represented throughout his hearings – he is capable and could have done it easily because he is used to giving evidence in trials and court hearings through his job – but you are drawn into believing you need legal representation and you end up in tens of thousands of pounds of unnecessary debt. It's unfair and unjust for some people. Until recently, people who were subjected to domestic violence were allowed to be cross-examined by their ex-partner, their perpetrator, if they were not represented by a legal team. I found that appalling. That you leave the person who has subjected you to such horrors; they're then allowed to stand up in front of a court and ask you intimate questions and make accusations about your answers when you have lived in fear of them for years? It is something that Women's Aid fought so hard to get removed from the family court system and they finally won. When I heard that news it made me so happy to be able to pass it on to so many of my warriors.

The Family Court system is better than it was, but it still needs improvement. Families continue to be let down too often and ultimately the decisions it makes affect children's lives for years.

After two years of hell we became a family of seven, the family we are today – but it was hard. We had fought for so long – the Family Court, social workers, CAFCASS officers, the school, family, strangers, friends, solicitors and barristers. We had to ignore the lies all over Facebook and were unable to defend ourselves. We lived in fear that Josh would be arrested again. We were unable to talk about any of it when the kids were around through worrying that we would be accused in court of not protecting them from overhearing 'adult conversation', so we did stuff by text, email or hushed tones when they were asleep. We got used to being verbally abused when in public while doing the school runs with the kids or in a supermarket.

Now it was all over.

We now were managing the boys ourselves – there were no more hearings, no more CAFCASS reports, solicitor's letters, and it was strange. It was hard to adapt to a life where we no longer sat under a microscope and we didn't have the constant battle we had been used to fighting for so many years – against everyone and everything. I still haven't got much of a life back for myself, which will seem extraordinary considering I run a page that has built a community of almost half a million people.

11

A HOME FULL OF LOVE (AND CHAOS)

It's hard to explain, but my life seemed to go from one shit storm to another for so long that it's had a lasting effect on the way I live now.

I have an amazing army of girlfriends who have been with me throughout the whole process but I don't ever go out to socialise with any of them – they come to my house. I feel calmer at home. It still feels odd to think we could go out if we wanted to. Since Josh and I have been together, I have never been on an evening out without him and I have only been for lunch once with my best friend Lianne and once with his sister Hannah. I have never stayed away from home without Josh. I don't go out of the county without him because my anxiety overrides it. In order for me to write this book, I have needed to attend meetings with publishers and agents in central London and Edinburgh and Josh has come with me everywhere. It's just something that I can't do on my own. I think it's because for so long, things were so bad that I didn't feel safe without him – now it's just a feeling I am used to. It's also what I am comfortable with. I am open and honest about that and my friends get it. They know I won't do girlie weekends away or girls' nights out – I've missed countless birthday meals and hen parties but they understand my reasons and so they no longer invite me along because it's just not me. They do know that my home is theirs, though and, when they come here, we eat nice food and drink wine and they know my door is always open. They also all love Josh, I suppose being raised around four sisters and his mum he is used to chaotic women, and so he gets it and a lot of the time my friends will sit and talk to him rather than me, about their shit relationships, their work or issues with their kids and he will chat for hours. Maybe in the future things will change but, for now, I only suppose I feel safe in my house with my babies and Josh. Other than him being a bird nerd when he goes to the moors or away with his friends to find rare eggs and nests, he also doesn't have much of a life without me. He could – I would never ever stop him or make an issue of it. In fact, sometimes I tell him to go and meet his friends for a drink or dinner but he refuses, I think it's just the way we have become because of the horrendous start to things. It works for us so we don't even really think about it anymore. Josh gets it, he understands why I am the way I am and I think deep down he loves me for it. It's just normality for us now that we are two peas in a pod and everyone around us accepts it.

Before becoming a part of my world, Josh and both his boys had led a really quiet life; the boys had never had friends round for a sleepover. Josh and his family tell me his home was almost silent. Many of my friends are like this – they can't be doing with other people's kids and craziness, but I am the total opposite. I don't do silent or quiet. I hate it. Recently during a therapy session my therapist asked if I could spend half an hour an evening when all the kids were in bed, with the TV off, in silence, processing my own thoughts and feelings and my first answer was that I was too busy, but actually, when we broke it down it became so clear that I can't. I don't want to stop running and slow down because then I have to think, as I have had to do to write this book. At times in life thinking hurts, slowing down to the point where the only thing you can hear is your own brain and the thoughts inside it can be utterly heartbreaking.

I hope that by talking about my life so openly, people might pick up on what might help their situation. Josh's boys had believed for so long that their dad loved my girls more. There was a lot of jealousy to begin with, and in some form, this can happen with any blended family. We sat all five children down and explained that it didn't matter who came from who, they were all the same, loved the same and treated equally and we were a family – a family that was now together 24/7 and a patchwork family that was going to be absolutely fine.

Due to Josh's shifts, I had to do the school runs each day from very early on, and that had its challenges too. Edie was at nursery and the boys went to school in a different town to Betsy and Tallulah, but had the same start time. I had to do three drop-offs and then get to work by 9 am while remaining calm. I worried about everything to be honest – even normal everyday stuff. I had been under the spotlight for so long from every authority and professional that I got myself in a state about disciplining the boys. I was overthinking everything. Seb had been through masses and some mornings with him were absolute hell. He was so angry at times that he was desperate to test me. My therapist explained he would do this to make sure he was safe with me, that I wasn't going to let him down, but he got me to a point that no other child has ever got me to where I would cry with anger when I was alone. At times Seb didn't stop until he got a reaction where I showed I was angry or upset, and while he went out of his way to get this reaction, life was at times unbearable for the other four kids. When he first came to us, nights were horrific. I couldn't settle him for hours and he would wake constantly through the night. If Josh was working nights Seb would sniff my drinks when I wasn't looking to check I wasn't drinking alcohol. To this day, Josh and I don't drink alcohol together if we are with Sebastian because he goes into a total panic that we will both get intoxicated to the point we won't be in control and something bad might happen. It's difficult to explain to him that for some adults it's normal to have a glass or two of wine together of an evening. I am used to this now; it has been almost three years, but at the start it all felt like a battle I would never win.

I would arrive to work late with puffy eyes because I just felt I couldn't cope and had sobbed the whole way in. Evenings were now a rush of clubs, cooking tea, cleaning up, baths, sorting uniforms for the next day, and making packed lunches. It just seemed so hard at times. I was drained . . . but then I would watch Isaac and Tallulah giggling so much together they were in physical pain, or I heard Edie refer to Seb as her 'big brother' when she kissed him goodnight, or one of the boys would just love me – they would come over while I was cooking their tea or folding their clean washing and wrap their arms around me for no reason at all, and I remembered why we were doing it.

I knew then why we were exhausted and worn out and skint – because we hoped that one day we would have five adults who would look back and remember a childhood that wasn't perfect but know they were loved – unconditionally – and even when we got things wrong, they would know we were trying our absolute hardest to get them right.

That's why we have a crazy house, I suppose. I don't really go out, so I bring everyone here, and I never want any child to feel unwanted or unloved. My nieces and nephews are treated like my own children and are more like siblings to my kids. The girls' friends are always here and, for some reason, our house is the one where the whole neighbourhood likes to hang out.

The boys had to get used to a chaos they'd never known before, as did their daddy, but it's a good chaos. It's a chaos in a home that's full of love. One where my friends let themselves in and put the kettle on and fold the laundry if I'm not home from work. One where their kids grab food from the cupboard or fridge and put the TV on even if my kids aren't home. It's a chaos that I created because of my own childhood, where I craved having a friend over but wasn't allowed. I remember lying in bed promising that when I grew up my house would be full of love and busy with people and that's what I've got, and it's something I never, ever want to stop.

Recently, Betsy's friend turned up having climbed out of her bedroom window while she was grounded. I answered the door to her as she was sobbing, and I told her Betsy was at gym but I invited her in for a cuppa and a chat. While drinking that tea and eating a pack of chocolate hobnobs between us, she took me straight back to my teenage years when she was trying to explain her feelings, where life right then seems so unfair, when parents are arseholes who don't understand you and think you're lying even when you're not. I got it, but now I am the parent, I also get how we live in fear that our kids are lying and getting into situations they don't need to be in. As I gave her a hug and wiped her tears, I reminded her that her dad does love her even though she's convinced he doesn't; he just wants to protect her and keep her safe and tiny forever.

It's so hard for a teenager to see it like it is; secondary school is really such a small part of your life, and it has such a small impact on you once you get into the big wide world where you might go on to university, choose a career, have babies, meet your future partner, but while you are in that secondary school, it swallows you up. It is the be all and end all of everything and it's impossible to see life after it.

I suppose with Betsy I am quite lenient, or maybe trusting – I allow her to go out with her friends, I rarely ground her and to date it's been fine, she's generally a good kid. She is the youngest in her year, as her birthday is in August. Some of her friends are eleven months older, and some in the school year above are two years older – so it feels like she has a huge age gap behind her friends, and it means, because of what they're experiencing, that I need her to be totally honest with me. I'm not stupid and I don't turn a blind eye. At the age of four-teen, I was doing things and getting into situations that now, as a mother, make me shudder at how it might have turned out. I look back and think I had zero guidance or support. I had no responsible adult I could talk to honestly or seek advice from so I make sure that my kids and their friends will always have that – they'll always have me.

I don't threaten Betsy that if I catch her drinking alcohol I will give her the worst punishments that will make her feel like her life has ended – instead, I explain the consequences. I make sure she reads the news articles where teenagers have got drunk and lost their lives because of their actions. I explain the difference in having a few sips of an alcopop to look cool in front of your friends but still have total control of your decisions and actions, compared to downing a litre bottle of Smirnoff and having no idea of what is going on around you.

When she tells me about girls in her year who are sexually active, I won't slag them off or bad-mouth them because that approach doesn't help anyone. No good will ever come from that at all. It isn't my place to judge or comment on any teenage girl who is choosing to have underage sex, but I can ensure that Betsy knows the dangers, the precautions, and I make sure if she is comfortable enough to do it then she passes this on to her other friends who may not, for whatever reason, be getting informed of them themselves. I explain how getting a bad reputation sticks with you and can be bad for your state of mind. I've explained safe sex and we have looked at every STD known to man on the Internet and Googled the images so she understands how gross sex is when you are not ready or responsible enough to be having it.

And that's all I can do. I'm not the parent that 'just hopes' my kids stay on the straight and narrow, I'm not the parent that naively believes my children will make good choices and decisions because they've been raised well. I'm not that parent because once upon a time I was the teenager who lied and stole and begged and borrowed. I was manipulative. At times, I was full of hate and anger towards the people who didn't deserve it – and despite me coming from a background opposite to what my girls have now, some of the friends I hung out with had the most privileged backgrounds. Some got dropped at school in brand-new limited-edition Range Rovers and lived in mansions. Some had mums and dads that I dreamed of having – but they still took illegal drugs, drank alcohol and had underage sex. They still lied to their parents and they still made mistakes, which is why I'm a firm believer that talking to your children, educating them, and making sure they know you are there for them is vital in helping them get through the most difficult years of their lives, no matter what their background or situation is.

●

Learning to live together is important, and I'm happy that my patchwork family home is now full of love and a lot of chaos. It's always a work in progress but from my experience, the following things help:

● Stick together with your partner when you're fighting the world. Try to see each other's points of view and when you can't, try not to fall out. If he isn't as strong as you want him to be with his ex-partner who you feel is ruining your life, try to see why – and if she is being an emotional wreck 24/7, understand her reasons. Life is hard when the world is against you but it's even harder if you're battling the only person who's on your side.

● Children don't ask to be born, they don't choose their parents or their situations, and they're just tiny versions of us. At times, we struggle to contain our emotions or stop our anger, so how are they meant to? If they've watched their parents go through a split, if they're meeting your new partner it's hard, because change is hard. They might become withdrawn, moody or angry, but you need to allow that. Allow them to express their feelings and just be there to love them, no matter how much they test you, because they're doing it to make sure they're safe. Deep down, all children want is to be loved.

● I watch, it's something I always do. I observe, and although my way of raising a teenager isn't everyone's cup of tea, I think, to date, we're getting it right. Keeping your daughter locked away from dangers like teenage boys and alcohol and walking the streets may work for a while, but teenagers are inquisitive and they like to rebel. They also don't open up and tell the truth when they know the consequences will be punishments for their foolish actions – and teenagers will be foolish much of the time, so if you can try and just stay calm, remember you were young once and just be there for them to come to you when they've messed up.

12

FIGHTING THE GOOD FIGHT

Josh and I decided to come off Facebook at the beginning of 2015. It had brought us so much negativity by the things that had been written and spread that we had stopped using it anyway. I sent one last post before I closed my personal account; it was the 'Shaldon Bridge' post to 'Spotted Torquay'. Within hours, things went crazy, so I decided to start up my own blog. The page gained around 200 followers within the first week and it stayed like that for a few months, gaining around 50–100 followers each week. There were days I panicked about what people thought about me, what they were saying and commenting, and I began spending my time worrying about people hating me for the blog.

One day, I had a really bad time and I was thinking about deactivating the page. Josh said, 'Why don't you write about it instead and explain how shit things have been?' So I did. I wrote it that night and then went to bed.

This was the post:

We are only into day four of 'back to school' and I've been a 'shit mum' repeatedly since Monday.

This week's epic fuck-ups have included:

Leaving two coats worth £60 on the pavement because I was too busy trying to convince a three-year-old it's OK to piss in a bush before we got back in the car. I remembered the next morning on the school run when we were getting bruised from the hailstones and I couldn't find them.

Had the morning from hell psyching Tallulah up for her swimming lesson at school where she cried (hyperventilating sobs where she nearly hurled into her Weetabix) from 7.15 am to 9.55 am that she didn't want to go, only to get to there and be told that her lessons don't start until May.

I gave Betsy no dinner money but only remembered at 2 pm when I was gorging on my own lunch at my desk, so I had a meltdown that she would either starve to death or be bullied for being poor.

Felt extra punctual and got the kids to school nice and early today – to remember on arriving I'd totally forgotten to collect my nephew on the way as promised.

I've done my usual – felt guilt, a load of rage and the usual feeling of being a totally shit parent; but then I thought . . .

A shit parent doesn't discipline their daughter before school for being an absolute horror then burst into tears in the car the minute you've watched her walk through the school gates because you think you were too hard on her – and meanwhile she doesn't give it a second thought for the rest of the day.

Shit parents don't stand in the rain in the freezing cold through winter every Sunday morning to watch their son play football, then reassure him how amazing he was for the whole journey home despite him throwing a horrific tantrum because he didn't score enough goals, while he's covering your clean car in mud.

A shit parent doesn't feel like they're failing because they've not read their child's school book every night of the week or practised their spellings and there's a chance they could have done better in that test if you had.

A shit parent doesn't sit in a meeting with a lump in their throat because they just couldn't get the time off work to wear a high-vis vest and help on the school trip to the zoo.

Shit parents don't feel shame because their kids have eaten McDonald's on a week night because they were just too exhausted to even think of what to cook for tea let alone make it.

All these things that make you feel like you're being a shit parent actually means you're an amazing parent – because you're doubting yourself.

Shit parents don't doubt themselves.

I've decided it's actually OK whether your kids are full of chicken nugget Happy Meals or roast dinner and veg.

It doesn't really matter whether they know the difference between 'their, there and they're' when they will learn. Remember, they needed that telling off before school – they'll thank you for it later when they have their own house and hopefully they won't leave their dirty laundry and dishes lying all over the place. One day when he grows up to be a father himself, coaching his son on a Sunday morning, he will remember that it was you who stood on his sideline.

So, this afternoon I finished work, I collected my kids – one of them then managed to put their foot through THE LARGEST pot of double cream in the back of the car. I drove straight to have it cleaned. I then had to try and explain to the guy (who spoke absolutely no English) that I had no money and try and make him understand I'd return after I'd been to the cash point – he looked like he wanted to end his life after looking inside the car and I had my usual lump of 'I'm about to cry with anger because my life is so shit' in my throat.

Instead of losing my shit, which I was on the verge of doing, I just thought fuck it – and took my babies to the cafe then we ate massive ice creams just before tea.

As I sat there with my double honeycomb sugar waffle beast with a flake, I decided, so fucking what that my car is going to smell of sour cream for the rest of the year? So what that it's been another week of kid drama? As long as our babies are fed, clean, loved, happy and not the spawn of Satan, most of the time we must be doing something right – let's not be so hard on ourselves.

I woke up the next day and had 80,000 new followers.

It was at that point I think I realised I wasn't the only parent who struggled. I wasn't the only one who felt like head-butting the steering wheel within minutes of picking my kids up from school and I wasn't the only one who sometimes felt I just couldn't do it. There were thousands of us – hundreds of thousands of parents struggling to cope at times. Most of these parents sent messages to my inbox as they didn't want to publicly comment in case their friends or family members saw and judged them. It was at that point I decided that I was going to just blog honestly about how fucking hard life can be.

The blog continued to grow and around June 2017,

after several chats with Josh and re-wording the post several hundred times, I decided to take a risk and write an open letter to a mum I was witnessing being subjected to domestic violence. I was passing her house most evenings after collecting Edie from the childminder and, one night, I witnessed a horrific incident where her husband/partner was trying to break into the house to attack her. When I saw her, it took me back to where I was all those years ago. I remembered how one time we got a letter through the door, Tony picked it up off the mat and it was addressed, 'To the wife beater'. It was a letter from our neighbours who said they were sick of listening to him and that he needed help. It said he was lucky his wife stuck around after how they had heard him behaving to me. He tore the letter into tiny squares then walked out into the street and sprinkled it all over the road while shouting as loud as he could about how people should mind their own fucking business.

I died a little inside that day, knowing that my neighbours knew what was going on – I was also ashamed that they knew I stayed despite what my children were hearing and seeing. As soon as I thought back to that day, I decided I had to help this lady. I called the police and Children's Services but the man remained at the house.

This was the open letter:

Dear petite pretty lady with the long dark hair,

I first noticed your house last year when I was driving past with one of my children.

You have a wooden and glass porch with another door behind it – there is a window to the right of the door, which I've decided is the lounge, and two upstairs windows. I pass your house at least four times a week on my commute home from our childminder's; I now pass it more just to check on you.

I noticed your house because we thought there was a man trying to break in – my child noticed it before me. He was smashing your porch glass with his fists and shouting in a fit of rage – it was only when I slowed my car down to look closer that I saw you and your two children behind the inside front door, screaming and crying. I wound down my window and heard him shouting the most horrific threats at you. I immediately panicked and pulled my car up into the pavement. An older man stood on the pavement told me he was calling 999.

I reassured my child that there was nothing to worry about and we drove home.

The next day I drove past your house with all of my children and saw you walking home – you were pushing your toddler son on his trike and your daughter was holding your other hand. The left of your face was black and blue with bruising, your eye was closed over, and you had cuts to your chin. Your head was bowed towards the pavement.

I felt sick.

A few weeks later when I drove past again with my children we saw you walking away from your house – your daughter was running ahead – with one hand you were pushing your son's trike and your other hand was holding his.

Your bruises had faded and you were smiling.

I felt sad.

I reassured my children there was nothing to worry about and we drove home.

The next week I drove past with my eldest daughter and saw your little girl in her pyjamas sat on the top step outside your house crying. It was freezing cold. I turned my car around and parked. I pretended I was just a pedestrian and when I walked past, I asked her in a whisper if she was OK. She didn't answer me, she just nodded her head in between her sobs to confirm she was and she ran in the house and shut the porch door behind her – only she left the inside door open so I could hear him shouting and you screaming, begging him to stop. Your toddler son was sat in the window. He seemed to have no expression on his face, he was just looking out towards the traffic.

I felt sick again. I called 999 and told them what I'd seen.

I called Children's Services the following morning and wrote a letter.

I then got back in my car and reassured my daughter there was nothing to worry about and we drove home.

I've since passed your house often – for weeks I see nothing, sometimes all the curtains are shut in the daytime for days. I worry you're not OK. Sometimes you are outside sat on the step with your children and sometimes he is there. I've seen you since with more bruises to your face. I have pulled the car up several times and just wait while pretending to write a report or make a call, hoping you're left alone and I can quickly run over and slip you my number on some paper so I can help you, but you're never alone and I am scared of your response.

You may not want my help.

Last week when I passed, he was down the road – I had to stop at the shop close by so I pulled up and studied him with the car window open; I don't know why – I just felt I had to. He made me feel so many things at once – sickness, rage and utter disgust.

He was throwing your son in the air.

If I'd never seen him before, I'd have thought it was so cute – I'd have thought he was one of the dads that the world needed more of.

Your son was squealing in delight ('More, Daddy!') and it looked the perfect scene. Only it wasn't.

Really, it's horrific. This baby boy is in awe of a man who is abusing his mummy, his sister and him. What is that teaching him?

Your children look clean, they look well fed and they're dressed really trendy and immaculately, always. I often hope I'll see them in their uniform so I can see what school they attend and I can help you there – away from him maybe – but part of me thinks you'll think I'm crazy and I question if I am being. I don't know what I would do if a total stranger approached me knowing details of my life.

I talk about you often, to my friends and family.

I think about you and your babies every night before I fall asleep and I worry for you every morning when I wake up. I wonder if there's a chance that maybe you haven't woken up and if you haven't, whether I should have done more.

I feel angry at you too sometimes that you stay in that situation, that you're not leaving to protect yourself and your babies – but then I feel a horrendous guilt.

I have no idea of your situation, your support network or anything else you're going through – who am I to judge?

My children often ask about you – and I lie.

I lie to protect them – that things aren't as they look and that you're actually fine.

I tell them your babies are happy and 'he' is probably a very nice man.

I then question myself – am I wrong to do that? Should I tell them the truth that I think this man is beating the crap out of you and your children are witnessing it? This could be happening to the girl they pick as their partner in PE or the boy they play bulldog with at lunchtime.

Should I make them aware that this abuse goes on in the world – every single day? That then makes me livid with him that that there are men and women who make me have to ask myself these questions and leave me not knowing how best to protect my own children because of the abuse they make others endure.

I frustrate myself at home – my fiancé is a police officer and when I rant at him he reels off the statistics at me. I know he's attended incidents where people have been so badly beaten by their partners they have broken bones and are left unrecognisable, yet they still lie to him for their abusers and are adamant they just 'fell down the stairs' by accident, even when they have their own children witnessing it – and they go back for more, time and time again.

Sometimes he wins and charges get pressed against

the abusers without statements from the victims and they get brought to justice – but sometimes they don't and I know some things he's seen break him a little inside too.

Then I question whose job is it to help? Why is nobody helping you? Or are you refusing help? Are you convincing the agencies that you're OK?

I've written and deleted this post so many times for the fear of it somehow reaching your partner and your life possibly worsening in some way. Then I think of printing it off and posting it to you when he's not home in the hope I can help you. I have stopped myself from knocking on your door so many times when he is home and letting him know that I think he's a hideous human being who's destroying his children's whole future and ruining your world.

What this situation shows me most is how extraordinary it is that once again somebody has made such a huge impact on my life yet you have no idea I even exist. I won't stop checking on you and your children and I won't stop calling the correct authorities when I witness his abuse.

And maybe this post will reach you, and actually instead of it destroying your life it might just make it better – which in turn means when I pass you in the street I won't be lying to my children when I tell them everything is fine – and

I will then go to sleep at night without my heart hurting for you.

Sending you so much love.

Within 24 hours of writing that post, I had so many inbox messages I couldn't keep up. I was being contacted by domestic abuse support services and women's refuges all over the country asking if they could print and share my post. I realised that domestic abuse was a huge issue within the UK and it touched me more than anything else I had been involved with, so I knew I had to help. As the messages continued to pour in, I started wondering how I could help these services. Yes, I had a platform to raise awareness but I wanted to do more than that – I wanted to help change lives.

I sat down and thought about the best way I could do things – I decided to begin by going back and personally thanking the women who helped me at the refuge I lived in in Exeter. I went online and called them. I was informed that due to government cuts, the refuge had been closed down in 2014. I arranged to meet the team at Stop Abuse For Everyone (SAFE), which was now a support service they had set up when they had lost their refuge. I spoke to Jacinta, the managing director, and I was heart-broken to hear how much of her job role was fighting for the funds just to stay open. She had lost many of her staff because they couldn't afford to keep them on, and the government was continuing to make more and more cuts while the problem of domestic abuse was continuing to worsen. I asked her what her service needed and she said they were desperate for craft items, which they used for trauma play therapy for the children who had been subjected to domestic abuse. Craft items . . . I shared their Amazon wishlist on my page and asked for support in buying gifts to enable the staff to continue to work with these warrior children. The number of parcels SAFE received was beyond anything we could have imagined. They were running out of space to store them and they kept flooding in. It was such a nice thing, seeing the impact of social media in real life. After that, I knew I could help to make an actual difference and I began to think of other things to do.

I decided to sell personalised calendars with pictures and quotes and some stories of what the page had achieved. I gave a chunk of the profit to different organisations, SAFE being one of them, and they were so grateful. We stayed in touch and a few months later I went on a course to train to do volunteer work for their service. Some parts of the course were harrowing. The videos we watched re-played in my dreams, and the stories we were told by the amazing training facilitator made me see that this was what I wanted – this was what I was here to do: to make a change to people's worlds that were being ruined by domestic violence.

We watched a video of one mum who upon leaving her husband had been frightened for her life. The police said repeatedly that they would speak to him and didn't. One night a few weeks later, he broke into her home and killed her, he then hung her on her own staircase in front of his tiny sons to make it look like she had committed suicide. He then instructed his sons to call their maternal grandma once he had left and tell her they had found their mummy who had killed herself.

That story devastated me. I watched her totally broken elderly parents try to tell her story, how they had been let down by the police, and how her sons were now being raised by their uncle and aunt because their father murdered their mother. I watched them explain that they had agreed to make this video to raise awareness for others. I found out that when you are about to leave or have left a DV relationship, you are at your most vulnerable – you are at the biggest risk from being murdered. At the time of writing, two women a week in our country are killed by a current or ex-partner. I found out so much about domestic abuse that I didn't know, even though I had experienced it.

I receive regular emails from SAFE with updates on their cases or asking me for help to raise funds through my page. The people who follow my page have donated so much, to so many organisations, that they have truly changed the lives of so many others, especially warriors and their children who are fleeing domestic abuse. I continue to help but it takes a lot of my time, and when it all becomes too much, I have to remember I am only one person. I get up an hour earlier each morning to go through new messages and check on the warriors I am supporting and I stay up much later than I should at night doing the same.

I am told by professionals I need more boundaries. I need to switch off, but the main problem with domestic abuse is these people have no-one – and the violence and control is so engrained in them that they fear if they contact the police or Children's Services, they will lose their children. They genuinely believe this, so they come to me, because I am the safe option. I sit in a little area where they know that I am not going to remove their children or give them a criminal record. I need to try to undo all the damage the perpetrator does, I need to be available to give them support, advice and reassurance. I need to ensure they speak up and get help because if I do switch off and miss a message it really could be a matter of life or death.

I also want to raise awareness of domestic violence. That's something I can definitely do through the page – and it's part of the reason I'm writing this book. Some people who haven't experienced domestic abuse believe that it only goes on between people who already have issues: people who are within the care system, on benefits, who refuse to work. They naively think these are the types of people that domestic abuse affects – and this is so wrong.

I remember when I was little and I used to visit my mum. She went to lots of houses over the years to clean and work for the super-rich. One of these couples had a huge home; he was a well-respected businessman in the town where they lived and his wife was a lovely, quiet woman, but sometimes she wouldn't be seen for weeks, and that's because he would beat the shit out of her – out of her whole body, her face, limbs, and she would be black and blue, and couldn't face the public.

I have sat in on Pattern Changing courses where the women attending are GPs; they are the doctors who treat our children for coughs and colds, yet these women who earn a huge salary are going home and being abused by their husbands – it is that real, it affects members of society everywhere. It doesn't matter if you're black or white, rich or poor, female or male. A domestic abuser is a domestic abuser, no matter what.

And I want to save anyone I can who is being affected by domestic abuse.

● Right now in the UK, 20 per cent of children are living with an adult perpetrating domestic violence. That means that one in five babies you see running round the school playground is affected by abuse. That abuse affects them, no matter how much you think it doesn't. Please, stay aware – and if you know about a situation of domestic abuse, report it. Ultimately, if you don't, the consequences could be deadly. By speaking up, you might be helping to prevent murder.

● Don't be frightened to fight for what you believe in. I fight against domestic abuse because it's in me. It's in me to help men, women and babies who are unable to help themselves without support, but some people don't get it. I have received emails on my page from people saying they don't want to read about domestic abuse because it doesn't interest them and I have lost hundreds of followers because they don't want to see it – but that's OK. I have learned that I am still helping and saving. I would rather have a much smaller platform of people fighting alongside me than a much bigger one of people who don't want to change something that's destroying the lives of so many people around us.

● One person. If you help just one person affected by domestic abuse, that's enough. If you get one woman to safety, if you buy her children some clothes and toys to start again, or if you help a man or woman realise what they are doing is domestic abuse, you have achieved more than you could have ever imagined, because to them you will always be their hero, and heroes are what make this world a better place.

13

PTWM BEHIND THE SCENES

Making a difference

PTWM doesn't just cover domestic abuse, it covers, well . . . pretty much everything. I speak about taboo things that other people hide away from and I try to build a community where we can help others and spread positivity. To start with, when I first received negative comments, it would keep me awake at night. Whenever certain newspapers ran one of my posts online, the comments people left on their website about me were horrific and I would obsess over them. I would sit for hours, getting angry and upset. At times, I would feel so annoyed that I was unable to defend myself against thousands and thousands of horrid, negative comments, but then Josh pointed out that those comments were there under every single article, no matter what the story was about! These people behind their keyboards had nothing better to do than wade in on these articles and write the most evil, disgusting abuse about a total stranger.

I also started to realise that every time a post went viral, it disappeared as quickly as it went crazy – and people forget the nasty comments. It took time, but now I don't care if people come on my page and call me a shit mum or a crap wife. Despite sometimes feeling exactly like a shit mum or a crap wife, I try my hardest and I love as hard as I can, which means that I no longer lose sleep over the opinions of people I don't know.

I also have lost people I do know, that I really loved and cared for, some of which are my own family. People sometimes don't like change, and although I tear myself apart with the things I don't and can't have right now – a mortgage, an owned car, holidays abroad – other people look at me like I am living the high life because of the success the page has brought. They don't see the amount of hard work and hours I put in, they don't see I am still the same me. I haven't changed. I am just busier – but it's a good busy and if my friend or family member was busy doing the things I am I would ask how I could get involved. I wouldn't turn against them while telling the world 'they've changed' or 'they don't make time for me'. My door is always open to anyone. The only part of my life that's changed is my need to bring about changes for other people, for organisations, which in turn will make this world a better place for our future generations to grow up in.

During my therapy sessions I have explained certain things people have done or said, people who should love and protect me as I do them, but who instead have gone out to destroy me and my therapist broke it down so well. She asked me if, before the success of the page, these people had tragically died, how would I feel? I replied 'devastated' and her response was 'This is no different. The way they have treated you, the actions they have shown means there is never any going back. They have made things so final by their choices and behaviour towards you and you are grieving. You are grieving for their loss the same way a woman grieves for the loss of her husband whether he tragically dies or he leaves her unexpectantly. A loss is a loss.' Those words made so much sense to me. I am determined to move on and concentrate harder on the people that do love and protect me. Ultimately, people, whether total strangers or close family, can be unkind, but that doesn't mean you have to be unkind back. That is how I believe the world will change: because of more brave people, like us, being kind.

The page now is a full-time job (although I have my non-blog job as well!). I continue to write about the highs and lows of life, I raise awareness for things that touch me, but, more than that, I feel that I have been right there while a community has been built – the amazing 'Part-Time Working Mummy Crew'. I'm so proud and humbled by the amount of support the page has received, and the amount of kind, positive people who use it to help others.

In March 2017, I was invited to attend the Towergate Award Ceremony at the Dorchester Hotel in London. Towergate had named an award after my page: 'The Part-Time Working Mummy Unsung Hero Award'. I had to pick three finalists out of hundreds of nominees for an award to be given to someone who went out of their way for others. My three finalists were: a girl who had been bullied throughout school including suffering a physical attack which lead to her having epilepsy so severe that her mum was now her full-time carer; an amazing lady called Hazel whose house had caught fire due to a faulty fridge and had burned to the ground meaning that she lost all of her possessions, her daughter suffered horrific burns, and her husband died in the blast; and my third finalist was a young boy aged 14 called Joshua, he had a brother with learning difficulties and his dad had a terminal brain tumour – his mum nominated him saying he had no friendship groups as his life was dedicated to helping to care for his brother, sister and father and he had taken on so much responsibility. The winner was Joshua, who turned out to be the most beautiful, loving boy in the world – a true king who was going through an absolutely horrendous time while trying his best to cope with it by being way ahead of his years. His story was utterly devastating.

The ceremony was great and I was hugely honoured to have an award named after the page; it showed how much we had achieved and that it was now being properly recognised. Now there are almost half a million of us – mums, dads, teenagers, women who struggle to conceive, men who have buried their wives. It's a page for everyone.

Recently, we followed the journey of Louise, a mum who wanted to raise awareness of breast cancer; she wanted no funds, just awareness to stop other little girls like her six-year-old losing their mummies. A while after we posted her story, Louise's brother contacted me to say she had passed away. She held on for her daughter's sixth birthday, making it through the party before dying that evening. She also left behind a devastated husband and wider family. The reality of me covering that family story so closely, in such rawness, made me hope that women will check their breasts, and if they find a lump they will go to their GP. It makes me hope that maybe because of this we will save a life, someone's, somewhere, and so I keep going . . .

Bullying

The other topic which had a huge effect on me when I did some research was bullying within schools. I read and watched stories of parents whose children had chosen to commit suicide by putting ropes round their necks or overdosing on tablets. I watched a mother appeal on TV after her beautiful son, Felix, had killed himself after he stepped out in front of a moving train.

One morning soon after, Betsy showed me a game on Snapchat called 'The Letter X'. It was a game where you were given a name then you had to insult that person, using the app, as much as possible and you remained anonymous. The things I was reading about girls who schooled with Betsy, girls who had come into my home and eaten at our table were utterly heartbreaking. They were being name-called for having spots, for their weight, their colour, their dress sense – it went on and on. I decided to write about this and the post spread. Betsy and I were invited on *This Morning* to discuss the game and online bullying and it soon became apparent how huge the problem is. ITV set up the campaign #ItsCoolTo-BeKind where children are encouraged to be nice to one another and I was delighted.

I remembered being at secondary school and how it felt when people were unkind. I once walked into my English class and someone had written obscenities about me all over the broken plastic chairs. Everyone was laughing and I wanted to die. They did the same on the bed in the medical room and on the backs of toilet doors. There was a girl in the year above me who seemed to get off on being nasty to people and I remember finding it odd how she was such a horrid cow but everyone was desperate to be liked by her. She would walk past me and shout 'Pizza face!' because I suffered with spots. No matter how much I tried to suck up to her, she just seemed to hate me. There were other girls too who were just nasty. They didn't give a shit who they upset, I don't know why that makes other kids like them more – I suppose it's fear.

Back then it was a relief to go home at night, just to get a break from it all. No-one called your house phone to abuse you so you got a night of peace. You could switch off and worry about it when you woke up for school. Nowadays, you leave the school gates at 3.15 pm and it worsens. Social media and mobile phones, when used in this way, can destroy our kids' childhoods and it's horrific. They'll be bullied if they don't have a phone but, when they do have one, they constantly see these awful things written about them, which means that they lose either way and just end up tormented by things they cannot control.

I continue to share stories of bullying that distress me and I'm so pleased to have been made an ambassador for Kidscape – they are an amazing charity on a mission to provide children, families, carers and professionals with advice, training and practical tools to protect young lives. I am working harder to campaign alongside charities to get anti-bullying ambassadors trained up and in every secondary school to tackle this issue and I want to see a difference. I have two children who are now at that stage of education, and are seeing this daily. I have another three who will be going through it so I want to know I have done all I can to make it better in the hope we see kids being nicer to one another because, ultimately, I can't bear to see children committing suicide due to bullying.

Every little helps

The hard part of all this for me is that I can't share everything on the page. Some weeks I can get over one thousand requests to share people's stories and campaigns to raise funds. I get emails from all over the world, from fathers dying of tumours to desperate mums trying to raise funds for their children as they have weeks left to live. I wish I could donate to them all, I wish I could make everyone's lives better and easier, but it's impossible. If I filled my page with campaign after campaign, people would stop reading the content because they also can't help everyone. I have come to the conclusion that it's better to help some people than none – and hopefully the page will inspire others to help people too. But that guilt still sits with me when I read a Go Fund Me page and see pictures of a family in torment over a situation they need help with and I'm unable to help because it's unfair to pick which stories are more important than others. So, I donate where I can and I apologise that I can't do any more and I just hope that, by what little I have done, the world will become a better place.

When I came off Facebook at the beginning of February 2015, it was because I had seen what a toxic, horrid place it could be. I had watched total strangers write, like, comment and share statuses and pictures about me, my partner and our children which caused devastating effects and I decided I hated the Internet. I hated how it had the power to destroy people's lives with what it could do. Now that I have been running *PTWM* for a while, my view has changed; because as much as there are still arseholes posting personal statuses about their ex-partners, as much as there are teenagers playing hideous games on Snapchat to bully other children, there are also huge positives that the Internet can bring.

This year we have got women into refuges all over the country. We bought a little boy a new bike when his was thrown into a river by bullies. We have helped children who were removed from their birth mother on an Emergency Protection Order, we have raised awareness and funds for cancer, domestic violence, baby loss and mental health. That's the power of social media – and what an amazing power it is when it's used in the correct way.

PTWM crew

Since the page began in February 2016, as well as shedding tears for horrid, devastating situations, I have wept tears of joy, I have laughed so much at people's comments, stories and pictures that my stomach hurts, and I have met the most amazing, fun, loving characters along the way that make me see what a kind world we do live in despite at times questioning it. I have come to realise that, when I am having a shit day, someone's is worse. We just need to be there for each other. If Josh has been selfish, someone else's husband has been more selfish. If my house is dirty, someone else's is dirtier. That's the way we work; we make each other feel better – publicly. More and more, I get the comments that read 'I have been a silent follower for so long but I had to comment . . .' and all of those silent followers are met with love, support and advice from other followers. When I sit and read it, I realise that other than my children, this page and the network we have built is my biggest achievement to date.

A real-life part-time working mummy

And I still work – part-time! I've remained with the same company that I was with when I was a care support worker. Some women balance working a full-time job and running a family and there are others don't want to work again – there is no right or wrong and it pisses me off when people judge. Ultimately, it's irrelevant if a mother goes out to work full-time, part-time, or stays at home if she's doing what's right for herself, for her children and her mental health. But we all struggle at times, and we all wonder about other women, and I think this shows when I reflect on the fact that the most popular question I get asked now is, 'How do you do it?'

I think that the Internet has a way of highlighting the best bits of your life on a blog and covering up the lows, no matter how honest and open you try to be. People much prefer a Happy Ever After and it's what everyone is looking for. I am now the happiest I have ever been.

I am 'blessed,' as they say, but still I struggle. Some days I get up and nail the housework, I take all five kids out for the day while Josh works, I come home and cook a roast and he walks in after a ten-hour day at work to me thinking I am Superwoman. Then we get the kids bathed and into bed and we cuddle on the sofa and I think, 'If it all went wrong tomorrow, I would be so grateful that I had this.'

But some days are an absolute nightmare. Some days, no matter how many times I clean the house, it still looks like a squat. Some days, I do everything with a ball of anger in my throat and I get irritated by things that yesterday didn't bother me. Some days, I tell the kids to entertain themselves like I had to when I was little because it feels like they only want to go out and spend money and when we are doing that, they're still moaning and clinging to my limbs. Some days, when I am driving to the supermarket, the thought of what to cook for dinner makes me want to cry. Some days, Josh and I fight for absolutely no reason and we don't sit on the sofa together, I go to bed in a mood wanting to argue more and he goes to the lounge with a bird book because he only talks calmly through stuff and refuses to argue.

And life is hard. It's hard whether you have ten kids or none.

We have difficult times as a teenager – it's the shittiest, hardest time of your life and no-one understands you and everyone hates you. Your parents constantly think you are lying even when you are telling the truth and you feel like the whole world is against you – even at times your best friends.

And then when you're through with that – welcome to adulthood! Being an adult is hard: having to choose careers, stay afloat, fight off illness, pay bills and just live each day with all its struggles.

But I think if we were all a bit more honest about how hard it is, it would make it all a bit easier because more people would admit their struggles. More people would offer support and more people would just be kind. The world would become a nicer place.

The worst–best times

Sometimes, despite the fact I spend my life fighting the voice in my head that tells me to prepare for a shit storm because things are going so well (and a lot of the time that little voice is actually right!), things just work out good.

In May 2015, Josh took me to Turkey for my birthday. We split the children between our mums and sisters thinking it would all work and we could have a relaxing break and go away together. At that point, we were in the throes of Family Court with both of our ex-partners, things were hideously tough, and we were beyond stressed.

We were due to fly out of Exeter late afternoon and Josh wanted to go into the city to get lunch first, which seemed like a good plan. We went to Café Rouge and he told me he had to nip off as he had booked a haircut. I couldn't understand why he would have booked to get his hair cut by a barber he didn't know in a town we didn't live in when he is the most finicky person in the world about who does his grade two, but, never mind. So, off he went. I sat in the restaurant for what seemed like ages and eventually I left to have a wander round the shops. It wasn't long before I started panicking as he had been gone way over an hour and we needed to be at the airport soon, but he wasn't picking up his phone. All sorts of scenarios went through my mind – mostly ones where he had died in a tragic accident – but, eventually, he called me back and we met at the carpark. His hair looked no different – the only thing that did look changed was his flustered, red, guilty-looking head.

He assured me he had got his hair cut – 'just a trim' – and we raced to the airport where I had anxiety butterflies in my belly trying to convince myself he wasn't lying to me but knowing full well he was. He might not be dead, but I knew he wasn't being truthful. We got to the airport as they were shutting the gate and made it on to our flight just in time.

We arrived in Oludinez to the most beautiful weather and hotel, spending Sunday relaxing by the pool ahead of my birthday the following day. Just before we went for dinner, we decided to call the kids and I pulled my phone out to find numerous missed calls from my mum. When I called her, she had received a message from Sam to say he was holding onto Edie until I was back in the country. At this point he had only just begun unsupervised access with her and hadn't had her overnight for over nine months. I went into a full-blown panic attack. Josh had never seen me have one and he started panicking himself, trying to hold me close to him, which was making me panic even more. I threw up all over the hotel room floor. Edie had a set routine at night, she had a doll which she couldn't sleep without, and she needed the label of her comfort blanket in her left palm. She also had a favourite juice cup that she had chewed a hole in that she always took to bed. Her dad had none of these things – it was all at my house. Edie had never slept away from Tallulah for that length of time and I was so worried she would think I had abandoned her.

I genuinely couldn't calm down.

Sam had just moved house so I had no idea where he lived and I was going out of my mind.

Josh, as usual, was more rational, reminding me that although we felt Sam was behaving like a bit of a twat, he wasn't a nasty twat, or a horrible one. Edie was safe, she would be looked after, and she would adapt until we returned home in six days. This sent me even crazier – that he would think this was all OK? I started screaming at him. Six days? SIX FUCKING DAYS? There was no way I could leave my baby in such unfamiliar surroundings for that long.

I couldn't eat that night and I sat in bed repeatedly trying to ring Edie's dad but he didn't answer. I was sobbing, thinking that she would be crying for us all. The next morning, I woke and it was my birthday. Josh was so sweet. He had bought loads of cute wrapped presents that I could use on holiday like bikinis and flip-flops, and the words in his card were so beautiful. But I was spending every waking minute Googling flights to get home. Josh said we needed to eat so we went for breakfast and he told me to go and get on a sunlounger while he went back to get the towels from the room.

I just couldn't stop crying. I was trying so hard but my heart was aching and I felt like the most selfish mother to have ever thought I could go away and leave the kids and think everything would be OK. When Josh came back, he crouched down beside the sunlounger at my side. I wasn't making any noise but he could see the tears running from under my glasses down my cheeks and he wiped them away with his hand.

Kneeling, he pulled out a box from his pocket and said, 'Rach, I booked this holiday for us because I wanted to ask you to be my wife and I thought it would be perfect. I am so, so sorry it's all gone to shit.'

I literally couldn't breathe.

Not for one second did I think this was coming. It turned out that the whole time I had convinced myself he had spent an hour shagging someone else or dying while we were in Exeter, he was running to the jeweller to get the ring. It was, at that time, typical of our lives. He had planned to take me away to propose thinking it would be the perfect setting yet I felt heartbroken and was desperate to get back to our babies. As well as the guilt I felt over them, I now had guilt over Josh – I couldn't believe this had happened when he was trying so hard to make me happy . . . and then I was beyond ecstatic because I was going to be his wife and I felt guilty for feeling happy. It was just the worst–best day of my life.

I decided we had to stay the week, we never usually got a break like this from the kids and Josh was right – no one was dying, nothing was that bad; it could all be dealt with and sorted upon our return.

●

- Always fight hard to make a change. It's so easy to hate what has destroyed you and I get it because I've done it – but actually life becomes so much better when you turn it into something positive. So, if your mum was stolen by cancer, go and fundraise to help prevent another mum dying from that fucker of an illness. If you have time, volunteer to help others; the peace of mind you get from helping others is phenomenal, it's addictive and it's life-changing for the people you are helping.

- Trust. Don't let past relationships or shitty situations stop you trusting your current relationship. Try to look at things positively if it's something you can't change. Don't obsess that your partner is shagging about when in fact he or she is doing good things for you, and don't be a bastard because your head takes over due to your heart getting hurt previously. Sometimes we can ruin a really good thing by crazy behaviour that invades genuine happiness.

- Take time, deep breaths and think, properly. Don't panic about something that seems so overwhelmingly devastating when actually, if you just break it down into tiny bits and talk it through with people that support you, and work out a plan, it will all level out and you will be just fine.

14

OUR PERFECTLY NORMAL LIFE

We got back from Turkey and life went on. And it has gone on in a way that everyone sees because I now make it my purpose to let as many women as possible know, through the page, that all of this stuff, the real stuff, is perfectly normal. We're not superhuman, we don't have perfect lives, but if we were all a bit more honest about it and as supportive as possible, then maybe it wouldn't seem so shitty during the dark times.

One day, just before I started writing all of this, at 4 pm, Josh popped to the barbers to get his hair cut that didn't need cutting. He returned half an hour later, kicking off that the website states their shop is open until 6 pm, the sign on the door states they should have been open until 6 pm, but they were closed. He told me he felt angry because he had to go birding at 4.30 am, he wouldn't be home until 7 pm, so it would leave him no time to get his hair cut that didn't need cutting in the

first place. He ended his rant with this beaut of a statement: 'I'm so fucked off, it's so annoying. I can't fit in
anything for myself because I'm already doing something
for myself.'

I smiled and walked out the kitchen to the bathroom to take the piss I'd desperately needed for the past
35 minutes but hadn't had a chance to have as I'd had
a kid hanging off every limb. On the way, I muttered
(loud enough for him to hear) that the only thing he
would be needing to do for himself if he carries on being
a selfish fuckwit is Googling 'one-bedroom flats' on
Zoopla.

Later that day, I attempted to explain to Seb about
girls' hormones and mood swings after he asked why
Betsy is always snapping at him. I told him he has all
this to come again with Tallulah, then Edie. His response
was, 'I'm so glad that when I get my hormones I'll only
get a hairy ball-bag and a deep voice. It's gross being a
girl, I'd hate to bleed forever and be in a bad mood for
the rest of my life.'

Yep, you've pretty much summed it all up there in one
sentence, sunshine. And here's the proof of it – one night
last week, I made Edie homemade lasagne for tea. She
spat out the first mouthful and refused to eat the rest. It
had bits in, it was too hot, it was spicy, it was yucky, and
it was disgusting. The next day, I sent the same lasagne
along to her childminder to be reheated in a Tupperware

pot. She ate every last bit, and, upon swallowing her last mouthful, said, 'I love your lasagne. Mummy's is disgusting. I don't eat it.' This kid.

I've got five of these – five tiny turds that I care for full-time. It is hard to plan a day out doing something they all enjoy together, all at once, due to the age gaps and it's harder at times having the day at home trying to entertain them all. I find the key is being organised and I would love to tell everyone I am but, in reality, a lot of the time I'm not. Seriously, though, having multiple kids you do have to be organised if you can manage it at all. No matter how tired you are at night, make the packed lunches, get the school uniforms out and in piles ready for the next morning, check their bags for letters that need signing, make sure coats and shoes are ready to go, because no matter how much you convince yourself you will get up an hour earlier the next morning to do it all, you won't. You will hit the snooze button and then, when you get up, there will be a gang war. Her yellow polo shirt will have disappeared off the face of the earth. You will have run out of ham while doing packed lunches and apparently everyone now hates cheese and you can only find his left school shoe. Everyone will pick up on your stress and start squabbling, which sends you over the edge even more and by the time you get halfway to school, late, you remember you forgot to feed the fucking dog – no wonder he's depressed.

It's always better to go to bed with a clear head knowing it's all ready to get up to and it always makes for a better day when you wake knowing you don't have to worry about stuff that can ruin the first part of it. But you've also got to remember you have it hard, it's a full-time job having children and, if you're getting it right most of the time, you really are a miracle worker. You need to get to grips with the fact your house will never be tidy; it may be clean but it won't be tidy – because trying to have an immaculate home while caring for tiny turds is like shoveling snow when it's still snowing – and the only person that loses is you; because your kids don't care if the windows have mucky prints all over them, the dog couldn't give a shit if the floor smells of Febreze lavender and camomile cleaner, and your guests aren't bothered if they have to move a pile of clean laundry to sit on your sofa.

The main thing that matters is that your house is full of love; and that's a hard thing to learn – because we'd all love a clean home, we'd all love to be on top of our ironing and have an empty laundry basket, but life is busy and everything could change tomorrow. I have got to the point where I've looked at people I've met through the page, who have just been diagnosed with an incurable illness or been left permanently disabled from a car accident, and I think if anything ever happened to me, I would want my children's memories to be filled with me singing stupid songs to them in the bath, losing my shit over who licks the raw eggs and sugar off the wooden spoon when we spend a rainy afternoon burning fairy cakes, and how I woke them up by smelling their toes when they're sleeping at night. I don't want to look back and think I didn't spend time with them because I was polishing the sideboard or bleaching the sink. Life is for loving your babies, not cleaning.

That goes for stepparenting too. Being a stepmum or stepdad right now is one of the most common parental roles to have, and it is without doubt one of the toughest. In an ideal world, you become a stepparent at a time where your partner's relationship with their ex is amicable, and you slot in, it's happy, you all get along, and everyone's priority is putting the needs of the children first, but in real life it doesn't often work like this. Stepparents get a tough deal, you're put under the microscope by everyone to do everything right and the minute someone thinks you're not doing that you're ripped apart, yet when you are doing it all right no-one gives you praise or recognition. If things go smoothly, you will take on the stepchildren and get on with your partner's ex, you will work together and the children will love you and you become a family, but we don't live in a perfect world and many parents get hurt when someone new becomes part of their children's lives. Rather than work together, they can destroy each other – and, quite often, these innocent children get destroyed too.

Children are capable of loving everyone. The way I've always looked at it is that Edie loves my best friends and Josh's sister. She idolises them. She gets beyond excited when she sees them and is always desperate to visit them. This doesn't mean she loves me any less. It means she is happy and I encourage that love. When they have Edie, they put her needs first – they make sure she's fed, bathed and looked after; this doesn't take away my role, it doesn't make Edie question it or make her no longer want me as her mum. The role of a good stepparent is no different – they are caring for your children in your absence but sometimes bad ex-partners still make amazing parents. If your baby has an amazing parent then I believe they should be allowed to parent, always.

Being a stepparent who doesn't have a good relationship with your partner's ex is hard. It's emotionally draining . . . and it's hard not to give up, so hard not to think, 'Fuck this' and pack up and leave, because when you are doing everything in your power to help raise those children properly, with love and routine, but get knocked back constantly, it's hard to keep fighting, especially if it causes issues in your own relationship. It's hard and it's unfair and at times it's a nightmare – but I am a true believer in time healing, and maybe it won't heal to the point of ever being good, but it will heal to the point that children come of age to see right from wrong. They will eventually make their own minds up, and they see who were the ones caring for them, who thought of them, and they see this whether it is their birth parent or stepparent.

When you're in the thick of it and things feel like they will be this bad forever, they really won't because children grow way too fast and, before you know it, everything becomes much better. Ultimately, these children are far happier when adults get along. Children hate confrontation, they hate being questioned about what Dad said or who Mum was with. They hate being in the middle of fights between grown-ups. I know this because I spent my childhood there and I have personally watched this a lot. It damages children, it makes them feel things and take on a burden and responsibility at an age when they should feel nothing but loved, secure and carefree. So, as difficult as situations may be, as broken as your own heart may feel, and as much as you want revenge, don't ever use your children. Don't withhold them against a good parent, no matter how much of a shit they might have been as a partner, because parent alienation is one of the cruellest things to endure, for both the parent and child.

Even if you are with the father of your child, motherhood is lonely as hell at times. Whether you have loads of friends with babies of similar ages, or you have no-one, it is still lonely. Mother and Baby groups are daunting and it always seems like mums go in groups – if you don't have a squad by your side, rocking up alone is scary. I am desperate to start a Toddler and Baby group – ideally, I would like to have another sprog to start this (wink wink, Josh), but, perhaps, in the meantime, I can borrow a few off the mums and dads that come along. I want people to be able to come alone without any fears, so they don't worry about what they're wearing or how they look, whether they will fit in. I want to walk out to the pavement and meet the mums and dads who are convinced they're failing and are too worried to walk in alone, and I want groups like this to happen all over the country – run by kings and queens who totally get our insecurities and fears as mums and dads and carers. Upon the flyers or website there would be reassuring words, because sometimes they can do the opposite to what they intend. So whether it's a young single mum who's struggling or a multi-millionaire mum drowning in postnatal depression, they feel reassured enough to go. When they get there, they're not glared at or whispered about. They're not ignored or judged. They are welcomed, they are loved and they are supported, because parenthood is as tough as hell and it would mean our worlds would be a much happier place if we could all just support one another.

Having a platform has made me aware of issues that are important to talk about. I am desperate to do more to help with bullying. A few months ago, I posted a funny ramble on my page about Josh and me having a Saturday night out. Within a few hours, the post had gained over 20,000 likes and lots of people were commenting with funny stories. However, what I also noticed, which surprised me, was the number of nasty comments on the post. Comments about how awful my dress was, how shit my make-up looked, how bad my hair was. When I looked closer, these comments were left by other women. Women who in their profile pictures were holding children, they were with children, all of them, and I just thought, how the hell are we ever going to teach our children how wrong bullying is when we do it? How are we ever going to stop children committing suicide when the women raising them, the women influencing their lives, are on a public social media page in front of thousands of people choosing to tear strips off another mum, another stranger that they don't even know?

It made me realise that bullying isn't confined to the school gates – it doesn't start and stop at a certain age. It doesn't just go on between children. This happens all over the world, it affects elderly people, single mums, working dads. It doesn't care what race you are, what religion, whether you are underweight or overweight. It is going on everywhere right now, affecting too many innocent people.

Adults at times are so vicious; they give the children they are raising the most hideous examples of how to treat other people and, unfortunately, these kids then go into school and do just that. But sometimes children who are raised surrounded by love, affection, peace and calm can also bully. Bullying isn't just done by the child who's been subjected to domestic abuse, it isn't just done by the child who was removed from her parents because they had neglected her. Bullying is done by any child, whether rich or poor, privately educated or not, and the key to solving it is to see that.

Recently I was contacted by a female GP. Her husband is a surgeon, they have a beautiful home, their children are privately educated, they holiday abroad. They have horses in their garden and drive brand-new cars. She seemed a really nice lady. She came to my page because she was heartbroken after she was called into school to be shown footage of her son along with two others bullying a younger boy on his bike. This boy was pulled off his bike, he was spat at, kicked and punched. They removed his helmet and took £2 out of his pocket and ran off. This footage was filmed by someone nearby; she was too scared to approach the boys but after they left she went out to comfort the victim. She took him back to his house where she was met by his mum. She explained the situation and was told that this boy, who had been savagely attacked, had just buried his own father. He was also autistic so was often the target of bullies.

This boy's mum got the footage from the witness and went into this prestigious private school after recognising the uniform. This resulted in three students being permanently excluded and a devastated mother emailing me asking me where she had gone wrong. Bullying is that real – it's in all of our children's lives whether they're the victim or witness of bullying or the cause, and it needs more awareness. It needs to be stamped out and children need to know it's not OK. I pray we get bullying ambassadors into all secondary schools. It's something I have campaigned for alongside anti-bullying professionals, and as soon as I can, I want to be out there, working in schools, watching children being trained to help others. I want nothing more than to see these changes taking place and the bullying in our schools disappearing.

I guess all of this started from guilt – and parental guilt is such a bastard of a thing to feel. It first hit me after I returned to work when Betsy was a baby. Before I went back to work her routine was quite good. She still woke through the night for a feed, which I was told she shouldn't be doing by the health visitor at the time. When I went back to work, I was out the house all day due to the travel times on the bus. I missed Betsy so much. By the time I got home in the evening she was beyond overtired but was so excited to see me that she got herself in a total state within minutes of me walking through the door. So I started cuddling her to sleep. When she went off I would lie her in her cot hoping she would stay asleep. I realised it was ridiculous but by the time I decided to go back to putting her down awake in her cot, she was well and truly used to having me get her to sleep so it was hell. Absolute hell. She would kneel against her cot and wail; she would sob huge fat tears that left me feeling like I was the worst mum on the planet. One night I heard her stop crying and went in to be met with her having fallen asleep on all fours, her forehead against the cot bars, leaving a huge imprint on her head. I felt so guilty I cried.

I bought books on controlled crying; I bought books on the best ways to settle babies, routines, the lot. Nothing seemed to work, nothing helped me. That feeling I had of my baby being inconsolable no matter what I did was an awful one, and it's a feeling as a parent that sticks with you, and what goes from you feeling like you've failed while you're falling asleep on their bedroom carpet at 3 am holding their hand through the cot bars goes on to feeling like shit because they've come out of primary school on their first day desperate for a poo having held it in because they didn't know how to wipe their own bum. That then goes on to the teenage years where you can't afford to buy your daughter the trainers every other kid has got and you worry they will get bullied because they're not seen as cool enough.

Parental guilt sits with you; every time your child feels shit, you feel shit with them. Every time someone is nasty or cruel to them, it will feel like they have been nasty or cruel to you. Every time they hurt, you hurt, only you hurt far worse because you are their protector and it's a hideous thing to feel guilt when you just physically can't make everything OK.

●

Some weeks I get a few hundred messages on my page, but if I write a post that people can really relate to, I can receive up to 20,000 messages in one evening. I have thousands of unopened emails on the page right now because I don't physically have the time to sit and open them. Instead I have an automated message with an email address for people to contact me in an emergency.

The emails I plod through contain various things – some people just send me a love heart emoji to thank me for the work I do, some want to rant about their lives, others offer to buy my page for thousands of dollars. The main emails I receive, though, are from women being subjected to domestic abuse, women and men who are aware that someone they know is being subjected to violence, or women who have had their hearts broken because their partners have been unfaithful and left them, leaving them with no idea how to continue. It's a hard one for me, that question, because when I do my usual crazy thought process of 'What would I do if I ever found out Josh was being unfaithful?', or 'What if he ever left me for another woman?', I genuinely don't know how I would survive. I have actually Googled 'Is it possible to die of a broken heart?' Of course, I would survive, I would cope, I'd have to, but that thought is enough to make me feel a few seconds of what these women have felt.

Most of them genuinely didn't see it coming. They were happy, they had a nice home, they had healthy children. They were in love. Then, all of a sudden, they get the news that their partner is leaving them for another woman, or they find out they have been unfaithful, and they genuinely, physically, do not know how to continue to function or cope.

I get it.

Every bit of it.

Recently I posted on my page details of my friend who has an idyllic life with her husband. They are wealthy, have healthy children, a beautiful home, nice cars – he is an amazing father and husband, yet he's just had an affair, a full-blown sexual affair that only stopped when his heavily pregnant wife caught him. Of course, he's sorry now that he's been found out – he doesn't know why it happened, says that if he could take it all back he would, claims that the 'other woman' means nothing and that it was just sex . . . but you don't heal from that, do you? It isn't possible for your brain to accept the person you love has done that to you and that you just need to forget and move on.

When I wrote about this, the post gained lots of attention – it got people talking in the Comments and mainly I was left saddened because so many women spoke about being in this exact position. Some were years down the line and their hearts were still broken as if it had only happened yesterday. What stuck with me though was a message I received from a beautiful lady who had an amazing career. She lost both her parents within a year of each other and, after becoming pregnant by her partner, who she told me was a really lovely guy and an amazing stepfather to her child, she embarked on an affair with a colleague. He was also married with children. She convinced herself it was true love, and that they wanted to be together. Only when she was 38 weeks' pregnant, her partner went through her mobile phone and found out what was happening. He was left beyond devastated – as was her son who doted on his stepdad. She told me that, instantly, the thought of leaving him appalled her. The thought of raising her baby with the guy she was having the affair with disgusted her, and she was left in turmoil at not having given a second thought to what would happen to her son or baby that was due.

Now she lives with the consequences – away from her partner who left her, and with a newborn baby. She lives with the guilt of watching her son grieve for his stepdad and her baby not knowing his own father properly, a man who has been left utterly heartbroken at that betrayal and will most likely never, ever get over it.

And there you have it – a whole family ripped apart and every single member of it left feeling like shit, apart from a newborn baby who has no idea how uncertain their future upbringing is. When I spoke to this lady, I saw that she is actually a really sweet person. Her job means she cares for other people; she is a nice, decent, respected member of our society – unfortunately, she has made some awful decisions, some dreadful mistakes, but she is still a mum, she is still a human being, and she still deserves to be loved.

Women though, right now, everywhere, email me to tell me they have just been delivered the news their partners are leaving them, or they have just found evidence they are having an affair. These women are heartbroken and, unless you have had your heart broken, you won't understand there is no pain like it. It feels like a physical pain, an ache that sits inside you and it hits you at times you don't expect, it's like being punched in the stomach and winded and it suffocates you.

I can't mend a broken heart, I can't make anything better. All I can say is that the saying is true – that with time it does get easier, but when you're in the midst of it, it seems so hard to see a way out, and sometimes a broken heart brings bad decisions because when you are in such a terrible place it's hard to think straight. You may get into another relationship that, quite frankly, you're not ready for because your heart hasn't healed.

The only way to get over a broken heart is to learn to love yourself again. It is such a hard thing to do. It's one of the biggest challenges you will ever face and, in my thirty-five years, three children from two failed relationships, and a shit load of therapy, it's something I have only just learned to do.

•

So, where am I at right now? The Facebook page continues to be as busy as ever. After spending eight months convincing a warrior to leave her husband, last night she fled in the night. I woke up this morning to a picture of them in a safe place, two children sleeping, with her being safe but scared out of her mind. I work on getting the police involved, try to get a refuge or emergency accommodation, and do my best to get her to safety and reassure her she will be OK. The emergency email that would receive a few messages a day at the start is now full each morning from women desperate for my help. I spend my days contacting agencies all over the country trying to get urgent help for the most desperate, frightened warriors and their children. I'm also trying to continue the fight against bullying. Hopefully, in the near future, I will be working with charities and schools to help change young people's lives.

And maybe we will have another baby.

All of a sudden, since Edie started school in September 2017, I don't feel done. It's the first time in thirteen years I haven't had a sidekick and I'm lonely. People keep telling me I will get used to being by myself, having 'me time', and maybe they're right, but, so far, I hate it – and I miss being a mummy to a really tiny turd, so maybe just one more, a mini bird nerd/PTWM to complete our huge/tiny army. Ultimately, I just want to continue as I am. I want to continue with this amazing huge network of people who go out of their way to change the lives of others, I want us to keep helping each other with support, love and advice, and I want to keep reading people's stories and comments on the page. I want to continue to laugh so much that it hurts.

I have honestly, right now, never been happier, and perhaps that's because of the page – because I have seen how other families have been ripped apart by illness or cruelty and it's made me see how lucky I am. I want things to continue as they are now, I just want what I have to never ever end . . . but, if it does, I have also seen that people survive – the page has given me a sense of hope which I've never had before.

I am so grateful for all the support I have received. Although I am the one writing the posts and covering the topics, you are the ones allowing me to do it. You have given me this huge platform, your likes, comments, stories and shares have kept the page growing – it's meant we have made a huge difference to so many people, and it's something I can never thank you all enough for.

I think we all know that things can be tough – but in life there are also amazing times. Times that create memories which you will never forget and that make you feel happy.

And I make light of the small stuff. The little things that make a day pass that other people will understand because they've been there too and we can just giggle together. I'll never run out of stories because that's what life is and I love that I have all of you to share them with. Last week, I received a call from the water suppliers advising me they were 99 per cent sure we had a water leak due to our ridiculously high consumption. Josh went out in the road and surprisingly managed to find the meter to undertake a leak test.

It turns out there was no leak. Just a teenage daughter who likes to ruin my life by using half the salon-size bottles of shampoo and conditioner every hair wash, spends 36 minutes shaving each leg, while singing along like she's some platinum-selling record artist, giving no thought to the water bill or the fact that when she emerges from the bathroom it's basically a sauna.

Josh called his usual family meeting round the kitchen table, warning all six of us that Christmas would be cancelled unless the water bill goes down. Edie was looking at him like he'd lost the plot, Betsy nearly vomited, muttered an abusive swear word and stormed out when he threw out the sentence, 'If it's yellow let it mellow, if it's brown flush it down!' Every night since, any time Edie hears the shower come on she has a full-blown panic attack and repeatedly screams, 'In and out, in and out, in and out.' Ideal.

That's our normal.

And that's life isn't it – I waltzed into Betsy's room one Monday with her clean uniform and, as I lifted her blind to wake her, she informed me she was on half-term. I threatened her with death unless she got up. She went crazy. I checked the website and found out she was correct and had two weeks off, which sent both her siblings into meltdown that they were still at school and me round the bend because she'd turned the house into a hotel and appeared to have forgotten to do everything from picking her dirty clothes off the bathroom floor to putting her Weetabix-cement-encrusted bowl in the dishwasher

– but it's all good because she now has a year-long streak on Snapchat, which has uncovered the fact that, every time I've banned her phone, her mates all have her passwords for her accounts. Brilliant.

I felt so sorry for the dog having to live in this house with all of us that I bought him a new bed and personalised toy box . . . and he still hates his life. When Edie and I attended Seb's Leavers' Assembly she met all her new teachers and friends' mums. As everyone was talking to her, she decided to turn shy until a lovely lady asked her if she had any brothers or sisters and she replied, 'Yes, I have lots, and I have a dog called Winston who can lick his own willy.' What a talent . . .

And that is my life. Me, Josh, Winston, and the tiny turds – and the hundreds of thousands who have made *PTWM* what it is.

And I think that's it. I am writing this last part tucked under a blanket while my babies sleep in the seats behind me and my husband drives us home from Scotland.

Husband.

That word is going to take some getting used to.

Yesterday we got married at Gretna Green. Just the seven of us. You see, as much as I have this platform where I gob off about anything and everything to thousands of people, the thought of walking down an aisle in front of people made me want to vomit. So, instead, we decided to come to Scotland with our five babies and get married at a famous landmark. And it couldn't have been any more special. Josh and I married in the most beautiful suite at Smiths Hotel, our minister was amazing and our children gave us away. We dragged in a couple of strangers as witnesses and we had a Scottish piper playing throughout the ceremony. Josh couldn't stop crying when the girls and I walked in and when I took his hand it was shaking like the first day I met him in his car.

And after we got married we had a meal together in a private dining suite where all the kids tattooed my legs and got off their faces on slush puppies and we then all jumped in the huge hot tub listening to Edie reciting *The Gruffalo*.

All the kids were sound asleep and, as Josh and I crawled into bed at 10 pm, he gave me the leg squeeze and the forehead kiss and whispered, 'I'd go through it all again'.

And right then I believed that sometimes you do get your happy ever after, and right now as I am sat in this car watching his hand on the steering wheel with his shiny wedding ring, I feel like I have won the lottery . . . although that feeling may not last because we're currently driving to Stoke-on-Trent to have a 'Familymoon' where we have booked attractions like Waterworld, so no doubt after spending 45 minutes chasing Edie round the toddler pool playing sharks or being made to go down death slides with Betsy when I can't swim, I will no doubt forget that yesterday I married the man of my dreams because normal life has resumed . . .

So now the page continues. We carry on as a huge army of help and I will carry on writing posts that some people hate but some people love, filming Josh topless when he doesn't know it, horrifying my kids when I give advice to the world, and just looking for those little bits in every day that make it all worthwhile.

My final bit of advice is to Josh – I really just want
him to read this, and to know that I mean it, and to
know that I couldn't be *PTWM* without him . . .
well, not this version!

Dear Joshua,

Your hobby has become quite famous on this
page. When you're now in public, women you don't know
shout 'Bird Boy!' regularly.

Between the months of March and July, your love of
birdwatching and nest-finding takes over. Any free time
you have, you spend on Dartmoor, leaving before 4 am
and returning at 6 pm on a massive high or a mega low
depending on how your day has gone.

In the past year you've travelled to Iceland, Fuerteventura
and the Pyrenees trying to find the rarest of birds.

And we fight.

We fight because at times I don't get it; I don't get why

you'd ever become so obsessed over a hobby and we fight because you try and reassure me it doesn't come before me and the kids, but at times I can't help but feel like it does. We fight because for five months of the year I'm doing this shit alone, and it's hard. I resent you because I don't understand it. At times, I'm envious because I wish I had something I loved like you do.

Tonight we travelled to Oxford, where you were invited to present a slide show of the rare birds you've seen and the nests you've found, to the most knowledgeable birdwatchers in our country. When you asked me to go along I wanted to say 'No'. These aren't my type of people, birds aren't my interest and I felt like I just wouldn't have fitted in, but in the past eighteen months, you've followed me all over the country to support this page; you've spoken to warriors in need of police advice and you've sat with me through the night when I've needed to work, so I agreed . . . and tonight I watched you give your presentation. I watched you talk about all the birds and nests you've found in the countries you've been to. I watched you show the pictures of what you've seen and I listened to your passion and love for what you do. The same passion and love your mum and sister tell me your dad had, that he instilled into you before he died when you were just twenty-one years old, of the cruellest illness.

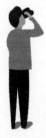

And as I listened tonight, I still didn't get it. I'll never understand what makes you want to set your alarm for 3 am to leave and go find the nest of a tree pipit in the middle of nowhere, but what I do get is how amazing you are. For the summer months you disappear, but you make it up to our family in the winter by being the most amazing dad and partner. You don't go out drinking, gambling or cheating, and you treat our family with nothing but love and respect.

So tonight, when I watched you be a bird nerd, you made me want to fight harder for what I believe in, because you took me on as a single momma when I had three babies 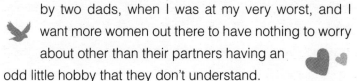 by two dads, when I was at my very worst, and I want more women out there to have nothing to worry about other than their partners having an odd little hobby that they don't understand.

I love you so much, I'm immensely proud of what you do and who you are, and you're hot as fuck.

Rach xx

ACKNOWLEDGEMENTS

Joshua – thank you for coming along when I was at my very worst, for healing my heart and loving my girls like you do. Thank you for showing me what an amazing, devoted father looks like and thank you for fighting so hard to make us the family that we are. No-one has ever loved and respected me like you do and I am so proud to be your wife.

Tallulah – those huge dimples melt me every time you smile. You are the kindest, most gentle soul and you carry angel wings that will go on to move mountains. I am ridiculously in love with you.

Edie – you are a carbon copy of your big sister Betsy. You are the happiest, cheekiest, funniest little girl we know, and despite being the tiniest, you are the leader of our pack.

My boys – you are the luckiest little boys I know. You have the most devoted papa in the world who would fight to his death to do right by you both. If you follow in his footsteps the world will be a better place. My love for you is as fierce as the love I have for your sisters. You are both amazing.

John – my big bro. My hero. Thank you for having my back, always, no matter how badly I've messed up. Thank you for never taking sides. You are the kindest, calmest person I know and all the good parts I miss in our dad are so visible in you. I love you x

Matt – no-one tells a story as well as you. Your giggle makes me giggle and, although we endured shitty childhoods, we endured them together and all those memories will never leave me. I love you so much, no matter what.

Sammy – for giving me all childhood memories I want to remember. Thank you for saving me at times without even knowing that's what you were doing.

Aunt Marg and Uncle John – for being dedicated to your children and to each other. For just getting it right. Together. Always.

Nana Ethel – I still miss your smell, the lines upon your fingernails, doing crosswords in *Take a Break*, and the way you kept your dark chocolate digestives in the

Tupperware pot in the fridge. I miss everything about you all the time.

Lianne – a true warrior, right from the very start when you shouldn't ever have had to have been. The person who calls me every day just to check on me, no matter what you're going through. Counting down the days until you meet your 'kindred spirit'. My best friend. Always.

Han – for being you. For all the gruesome links. For explaining things to me in a way no-one else can so that life makes sense again. For supporting Josh and me through the most difficult years. For being the most devoted Auntie and for reminding us that we could make the impossible possible, and for getting your happy ever after – Grandfather would be proud.

Mummy Marshall – for still smiling, although life always seems to be against you. Despite learning to live with a broken heart after Richard died, you continue to do nothing but live for all of us and our babies . . . and you bake the best brownies.

Jo – for being the kindest, most calming friend there is. You are an amazing momma and one of the most beautiful souls to have entered my life.

Mel – for just making it work, with a tiny baby, away from everything and everyone you knew. I am in awe of you and can't wait for the day I repay the favour with a surprise visit to the Gold Coast.

Bex – for being the most devoted mum to Lils and being the coolest non-related Auntie to all my tiny turds. No, Betsy's still not allowed to get her nose pierced.

Leila – for going on to do amazing things and achieve the most successful career. I remain in shock you can drive a car through central London traffic. Stay in touch with me, always.

Kate – the most devoted mum despite having to fight daily. A fight I know in my heart you will win.

Kel – thank you for being the best mum to my niece and nephew, for always thinking of their wants and needs when times are tough. And for being funny – not as funny as me though. And drinking all my coke.

Josephine – your loyalty to me and my family is fierce and I know what our friendship means to you. Never forget what an amazing momma you are to your baby boy, and don't forget your worth.

Han – for always staying in touch across the miles, never forgetting my birthday, accepting I'll always forget yours and being proud of me always. I miss you.

Keith and Net – for being a part of our family and for looking after us, all of us, especially Winno.

Elsie – I feel sorry for the memories we talk about. I am beyond proud of how hard you work and I have no doubt you will go on to achieve amazing things, baby.

Mia – The strongest momma I know after enduring the birth and complications you had. The day I walked into that hospital ward and saw you, I broke; but you carried on, milking your boobs through frightened tears. Your beautiful son (and baby bear on his way) will one day be so proud of you, as I am.

My nieces and nephews . . . There will be times your mums and dads will piss you off and ruin your lives, I may not be able to make it better but I will try – because at times they pissed me off and ruined my life too . . . my door is always open and I love you all, so very much, no matter what.

Gayle – for answering that email and everything you've ever done since. My babies really love you.

Tracy – for looking after me when I was a broken 14-year-old and being the best mum to Rudi. I still have everything crossed that someday, somehow, you will get your baby, because no one deserves to be a momma more than you, you're the best.

Simone – for sorting this, and other things (including my life) most weeks. Rocking the shit out of being a single momma even when you think you're failing. You are simply, the best.

Stace – I knew one day you would get your happy ever after and despite you right now not knowing which son is which or having no clue what day of the week it is you are so lucky to have Dave and your boys, as are they to have the most devoted momma and fiancé ever.

Emma – thank you for giving me this opportunity, for your support and for believing in me. I am honoured to be a part of your publishing house.

Dave – for all the dodgy poems, the shit wedding present and your amazing giggle. I am so glad I was 'the' blogger that answered your distribution email.

My crew – to all of you. For the stories, comments, posts and pictures. The support and love you show me and each other blows me away daily. Together we have made changes I never thought were possible. I can never thank you enough.

Gabriella – the last, but one of the most important people in my life. I have never felt pain at someone else's pain like I have with you. Next time you are faced with 'that' decision, please remember I could never live without you. I love you.

THE BEST OF THE BLOG

I post lots online – rants, positive messages,
funny things, appeals for help and much more.
These are a few of the ones that have really
struck a chord:

EDIE & JUDE

On Friday, my friend arrived from London with her son Jude to stay for the weekend; ten minutes after my daughter Edie had met Jude, she needed the toilet. She shouted down the stairs, 'Mum, I need a poo but it's OK, Jude will turn the light on and wipe my bum for me.' He followed behind her repeating, 'sure', in his little Cockney accent. At bedtime, Edie asked him to have a sleepover in her room and his mum and I secretly listened at the door to their conversation:

Edie: Night Jude. Don't worry, there aren't any spiders in my room.

Jude: Night Edie. It's OK, I'm not scared of spiders.

Edie: I am, but you're here so I'm OK. I love you.

Jude: I love you too.

It made me wonder at what age we start to complicate friendships. We receive a text message without kisses, and question if our friend is being shitty. We are 100 per cent sure our friend has been shitty because of the tone of another text message. Our friend gets shitty because the tone of our text message wasn't meant like they thought. Our friend doesn't contact us as much, and despite us knowing they've got the pressure of children or a job, or both, we still convince ourselves we've lost an amazing friendship. We get funny over who our friends are friends with and rather than support each other over our choices of relationships and our decisions, we tear each other apart. We let each other down and at times things are said and done that become irreparable. Because of our broken friendships, it stops us entering into new ones because we fear getting hurt again, so instead of falling in love with new friends we distance ourselves.

So, as I sat on the edge of the bed and watched them sleep I thought, wouldn't the world be a nicer place if we all kept uncomplicated friendships for life, which started by wiping each other's bums after 10 minutes and an hour later we're falling asleep together whispering 'I love you'?

BEHIND IT ALL

Imagine your husband loving you so much. Imagine him constantly telling your friends and your family how much he loves you, kissing your forehead and telling everyone what an amazing mother and wife you are. Both of your social media portray a perfect family that your friendship groups are in awe of. Imagine that husband beating shit out of you behind closed doors, covering every part of your body that people don't see in bite marks and bruises, and slicing your skin open. Sexually assaulting you most nights once your babies are fast asleep but making you believe this is totally acceptable because you married him. Getting your wages paid into his account and him even filling your car with petrol so you don't need any access to the money you've earned.

Imagine being that wife, so frightened that if you speak up everyone will think you're crazy, including your beautiful, kind parents, because they all think your husband is such a good guy, dedicated to his wife and children.

Imagine having no support network and having your phone bills monitored so in the end you contact me, a total stranger.

And, after months of emails you send me the images of the damage to your body as it happens, so you can delete the evidence and I can save it. I convince you to speak by email to one of my warriors currently under police protection to share her story with you, and between us we build you up to confide in a work colleague. That work colleague took you to her female GP, a hero in disguise, who booked you an emergency appointment with a domestic abuse service which she personally drove you to in her car – and then you saw your support network was so strong that you are now actually invincible, and by talking to people you have learned that what you've been subjected to is not OK just because you took your wedding vows.

And then you took your babies and you fled, far, far away to a safe place.

And it turns out everyone you thought wouldn't believe you did, because actually, they saw your husband for what he was the whole time he thought he had them convinced; they just didn't raise it with you because in our society this isn't something we talk about – and how very devastating is that?

To everyone on this page helping me fight this fucker of a fight, thank you.

One day we will win and our babies will grow up in a nicer, kinder, safer world

BEING A STEPPARENT

I get messages daily asking me 'how I do it'. People wondering how our patchwork family always looks so rosy.

Let me tell you how . . .

Once upon a time I was a four-year-old girl who became another woman's full-time stepdaughter. I felt like I wasn't wanted.

My siblings and I would sob because we missed our mum; my brother and I would repeatedly have night terrors. I don't recall being hugged or kissed by our stepmother, nor do I remember hearing the words 'I love you' from her.

I felt that we were treated differently to her biological children who we had to watch come in and take over our family home. Her biological children who, looking back, were probably as confused as us at why their mother suddenly gained four new children.

I grew up with a broken heart and once I became a teenager, that broken heart turned to anger, and I rebelled. I rebelled so much that by the time I was taken into foster care, I was so broken I didn't understand how I should think and feel anymore. I rebelled as a teenager by taking Class A drugs and going to raves rather than revising for exams, and instead of sitting those exams, I got involved in underage relationships with older men under some illusion I would receive the love that by then I desperately craved.

I rebelled so much I ended up making many life mistakes that sometimes I am amazed I'm still here to write these posts.

I remember being laid on my bottom bunk bed as an innocent five-year-old, and being laid in a pull-out bed in my foster home as a damaged fifteen-year-old always making the same promise: that whatever children I ended up having in my life – be it step, foster or biological, whether it was my nieces, nephews or family friends' babies, I would love them. I would always show them love and affection, no matter what.

So that's what I do.

At times, being a stepparent is the hardest, most challenging job in the world and I get emails every single day from men and women who feel they can no longer do it.

There is no time for that honeymoon period you would get in a relationship where there are no children. The honeymoon period where you spend days and days together doing what you want, when you want, because there are already tiny humans that you haven't even met that come before you. We then go on to raise children who at times are hard work, who love to remind us we are not their real mum or dad. We can feel as if they truly hate us and go out of their way to cause us nothing but upset and heartache.

You can also have huge issues with your stepchild's biological parent which, in itself, can bring massive problems into your relationship.

If you have your own children, at times you can feel like they come second-best and you feel guilt towards them when you feel you are getting it all wrong.

We are being watched and judged on how we do things and the minute we make a mistake, we are crucified. We feel taken for granted and, ultimately, as stepparents we don't get any recognition that actually, we're doing a good job.

But hang in there, because despite these children constantly driving you crazy, despite them testing your patience daily and despite them treating you like shit at times, it will be worth it in the end. They grow so quickly and start to see things for how they were, maybe not straight away, and maybe they will struggle to admit it, but they will see the real picture.

They know who was there for them and who wasn't. If they have a biological parent telling them untruths about you that they believed as a child, they will grow to see this. They remember who spoke badly of others in front of them and who didn't, and they remember who loved them at the times when they were difficult to love. They will remember who treated them fairly with the right kind of discipline and who didn't.

Although I may make it look easy, I understand it's not.

I get that my approach isn't for everyone: it's based on my childhood and the things I've seen and heard and the way I have felt.

There is no 'step' or 'halves' in our household. The five children who reside with me right now are loved equally whether they came from my womb or not. Betsy and Tallulah have three older sisters who I helped raise alongside them for ten years and they will always be their sisters, not 'step', not 'half', just sisters.

Ultimately they are children. Children who were born into this world and didn't ask for the situations they've been given; they didn't ask to gain a stepparent, and as difficult for us as it is at times, and it is, it's also difficult for them.

All these children need is a little help, a little hope, a load of love and someone who believes in them, no matter what.

OPTIONS

On Thursday night I went to Betsy's school options evening where we met all the teachers and spoke about her GCSE subject choices.

I watched so many parents 'tell' their children what subjects they'd be taking, informing them what they need to study to do well in life and I've been thinking about it every day since.

I understand we all raise our children differently, but ultimately we all want to reach the goal that is best for them. I am not 'that parent' who is ever going to tell any of my children what subjects they're expected to study.

I'm not that parent because I hated learning, I suffered with horrendous anxiety when I didn't understand certain things, and I left school without taking any GCSEs so I had nothing but zero qualifications and bad memories. I immediately went into full-time work because the thought of learning in a classroom setting at college or uni gave me those same horrid feelings. Despite not doing well at school I've gone on to have a senior management role and I've always worked hard for what I have.

I am not that parent because I don't believe that for a child to succeed in life, they have to succeed in the classroom first.

Betsy trains at the gym most weeknights and every

Saturday; when she's not training she's volunteered to be a Young Leader at her gym. Her coach emailed me recently to tell me how pleased everyone at the gym is her achievements. Instead of going down the park with all her mates or hanging out down the beach in the summer, she is spending hours and hours helping other children improve their skills and in a year's time she will sit her exams to be a qualified gymnastics coach so she can do something that she loves.

Seb trains every night at football; he never spends his weekends with his friends and he has accepted the fact he doesn't have late nights like everyone else because he's chosen to travel all over the country playing matches against other teams. He has been presented with a Hero Award in his school for excellent captaincy and respect. After the award was given, his teacher stopped us to say he is the loveliest, kindest boy, and when the keeper from the other team was knocked down twice, he pulled him up and shook his hand.

That's what makes me see that my children will succeed in life.

And I am not that parent because seventeen years ago when I left school, social media never existed. We had never heard of it, it was alien to us; it is now something that has made people billionaires. Millions of people all over the world have made careers and fortunes from something that was not around when I was leaving school. I have no idea what careers will be available when my children are of the age to be making choices and going into work. I imagine they may be successful at something that doesn't even exist right now, so next week my eldest child has to choose her GCSE subjects and it will be just that, her choice.

INTERNATIONAL DAY OF THE GIRL

Yesterday I received a call from Betsy's Head of Year. She told me she was calling with good news, which makes a change – usually it's to inform me her skirt's too short or she's arrived at school late despite leaving from home on time.

I started thinking, perhaps for the first time, that she hadn't burned her ingredients in Food Tech, or she had secretly completed an amazing homework project I didn't spot, or maybe she had received fantastic marks for working so hard in class.

No, what Betsy had done was wade through a massive crowd of people where one girl had been circled, alone, while another girl was threatening to beat her up.

Instead of joining this huge mass of teenagers that were cheering this girl on to hurt the other one, who by now I imagine was petrified and had no means of escaping the ring of people who had circled her, Betsy pushed her way through to the front while screaming to everyone that this was bullying. She took the girl by the hand and led her through the crowd to the Head of Year while being called a rat and a snake by other children who were desperate to witness a thirteen-year-old girl get the shit kicked out of her.

My heart sank upon hearing the news and I told the Head

of Year she has a job I would never want and I questioned how and why our children are so cruel to each other. Questions, which as hard as she is working, she struggled to answer.

I know my daughter. I know that yesterday she would have walked into that crowd with her heart in her throat, her face would have turned scarlet while she was being abused by her peers for stopping something that shouldn't have been taking place and she would have been physically shaking, but she still did it – she didn't worry about whether she would get beaten up for intervening, she didn't think of the repercussions to herself.

I have thought about this all day today while worrying about how she's getting on at school and I've realised that actually, I don't care if she's a crap cook – it's not going to destroy her life if she gets a few detentions for missing homework, and ultimately if she doesn't leave school with amazing grades there are always other options. Give me a phone call like yesterday's any day, where I know I am raising a Baby Warrior who protects and loves others without question, because that will get her further in life than any GCSE or cooking degree.

I love you Bets, so much, and I pray you'll always be that girl who stands out from the crowd.

THIS WEEK

This week I have been supporting my friend. She is pregnant with her third child and, upon coming home early from a trip away, caught her husband having sex with his 19-year-old colleague. Upon checking his mobile phone, something she'd never felt the need to do before, she found out it was something that'd been going on for three months.

She idolises her husband, he idolises her. They are happy – they planned this third baby – they have a beautiful home, good jobs, and they love the two children they have together to death.

She is now left devastated, she has kicked him out but desperately wants him back. He is sorry, it was a mistake, but he has no answers as to why it happened. He has no answer as to why he had sex with another woman while his wife was carrying the child he desperately wanted. He has no answers as to how his other two children will ever recover from their family home being totally shattered and having to watch their momma cry, day and night. He has no answers as to how they get over this shit-storm of a situation and where they go from here.

People have affairs. They fall in love with people they're not meant to. It's life. It happens, and when relationships are desperately unhappy they fall apart, and sometimes someone else is involved, but, ultimately, everyone moves on because they know they weren't right together.

But you know what sucks? It's when people just fuck around for fun, when they're not actually unhappy, they're just bored. Because hearts get broken – the hearts of children. And people who have their hearts broken sometimes don't recover. They hurt, and it's a physical hurt where having tonsillitis for a year would be a better feeling.

So, if someone takes your eye and they are already taken, or if someone takes your eye and you are already taken, just admire them from afar and keep going how you are – back to the family, which, deep down you love, because actually, boredom isn't unhappiness, it's just a way of telling you to make more effort with the people who love you.

MY FRIEND

Dear X

Last year I began receiving emails from a woman who was being subjected to domestic abuse. The details of her emails, from a false account, were so horrific I prayed it was a hoax.

After some time it became clear it wasn't. She ended up being rescued by the police, close to death.

Other than me, she had no-one. She told me all about you, her best friend, who she had been stopped from seeing by her perpetrator five years earlier.

I spent hours tracking you down on Facebook and after finding you through messaging your mum and friends, I sat down and composed one of the most difficult emails I have ever sent.

I contacted you to explain what had happened to your best friend, your best friend who you graduated from uni with, and I gave you her address, where she was staying – under police protection, hundreds of miles away from you.

Without question, you got in your car and drove through the night, hours and hours to be with her. I know that upon getting to her that evening, the sight you were met with will never, ever leave you. You arrived just after she had slit her own throat open and you immediately got her to safety.

She remains, to this day, in hospital.

Both you and I are now her next of kin, and, as much as I help from afar, I can only do so much. Josh speaks to her daily to reassure her from both a male and police perspective that this world isn't as dark as it seems right now but you are the one doing all of this.

You are the one who has held her hand through countless operations; operations where experienced surgeons have left theatre in tears because they have never seen such damage caused to a human by another human.

You have been the main port of call for her liaison officer, who, ahead of the impending trial, has told you details of the case that when you have repeated them to me have made me physically sick.

You've read the reports from professionals which look like something out of a horror film. You have been there, day and night – washing dirty clothes, making her favourite food, buying anything she needs without question and doing everything in your power to convince this warrior she has something to live for.

And we aren't there yet. We get weekly calls from her ward: the suicide attempts are still there, albeit less often, the self-harm is horrific but still, we are trying.

I don't think in the past nine months we have gone a week without one of us crying to the other, without us getting those missed calls from the ward and phoning each other before we call back thinking that this will be the call we've been dreading.

And a lot of the time you are treated like shit because when someone feels they have nothing to live for, and when someone doesn't want to remember how lovely their life was before it went wrong, they blame the person reminding them, which is you. But you hang on in there – you fight, you fight with everything you have to keep this warrior alive, to one day get her back to who she was before domestic abuse came along and stole her entire being and every single day I am in awe of how you do it and keep going.

On top of that you have your own worries – and you have one of the most responsible job roles in this country working as a deputy sister in one of the busiest paediatric critical care wards, making life and death decisions over people's tiny babies every day, nursing the most poorly of children to their deaths and going home at night praying a miracle happens so when you return the next morning others will still be alive.

So, thank you for accepting that message request from me all those months ago, thank you for taking on a role I would have never been able to and thank you for saving a life, because I know without you being there that that first suicide attempt would have been successful and today this letter content would be very different.

I am so pleased to call you a friend. I love you very much.

Rach xx

THE LAST LAUGH

Last but definitely not least, here are some comments from followers that have made me literally cry with laughter. All of you brighten up my day, and I'm so thankful I get to hear about the hilarious things that happen to you (and we all know we are not alone!).

On driving while wearing flip-flops because your toddler insisted on your footwear style:

One slipped off. Cue panic . . . she rammed into the car in front. No one hurt, just a few dents. I can just picture this manic mother in mid-January doing the school pick up in winter woolies, hat, coat and fucking flip-flops because your three year-old said so.

On careers advice:

My 16 yr old who wants to be a heart surgeon btw asked if we were in the United Kingdom . . . I've told her if my heart stops to fucking leave me alone.

On potty training:

My daughter wrapped up her own shit as a present because I told her it would make me happy if she didn't poo in her nappy.

On sex education from an 8-year-old:

While eating our coco pops this morning. . . [he asked] me why did I let Daddy put his 'Venus' in my 'Par-Gina' to make a baby it's disgusting!

On techniques to settle a 2-year-old (who is scared of fart noises):

We have purchased a whoopee cushion and every time she moves from her bed it farts. All I can hear on the monitor is 'parp' followed by 'no no no fart! *Whimper* It's fine, it's fine'. She's staying put.

**Join the PTWM crew
and share your stories of
#APatchworkLife**

f facebook.com/PartTimeWorkingMummy

@parttimeworkingmummy

@PTWMUMMY